HOW GRAY IS MY VALLEY

*Enlightened Observations
About Being Old*

SHARON JOHNSON, M.S.

How Gray is My Valley
ISBN 978-1985065086

Printed and bound in USA

To my beloved husband, Howard Johnson.
You will meet him in these pages.
You will come to like him.
Maybe even love him a little.
But not as much as I do.

ACKNOWLEDGEMENTS

The most endearing comment I receive from those who have followed my newspaper column over so many years is: "It always feels like I'm having a pleasant cup of coffee with an old friend." In response I would say, "Thank you."

I hope this compilation of my personally favorite columns engages, educates, informs and entertains. That is my objective. I want readers to embrace healthy and active aging with laughter, or at least a smile, and come to recognize that aging offers many small adventures.

I envision you having fun with this book. Gift it to a friend. Read it out loud. Read it with your friends or neighbors or in a book club setting—coffee and tea optional. All the proceeds from this publication will go to the non-profit organization my husband and I started several years ago, specifically our "Grandma's Porch" Fund that provides assistance to low income older adults who want to safely age-in-place.

I thank and acknowledge all the members of our non-profit organization's Board of Directors, specifically John Bowling, Ellen Waldman, Paul Westerman and Vicki Schmall who encouraged me to keep writing in support of a healthier and stronger community. Vicki Schmall is one of several layers of editors I used in completing this book and I thank them all; but Vicki was the most rigorous. She was a kind and critical reader. This book is better because of her.

I greatly appreciate the Mail Tribune editors of my Healthy Aging column over the years, Bob Hunter, Cathy Noah and David Smigelski.

They allowed me to write boldly and without hesitation and supported syndication of my column.

I thank and acknowledge Maggie McLaughlin who introduced me to self-publishing and paved the way for this book to actually happen. If you have a book in you—Maggie can help you exit it to the printed page.

I especially thank my incredible husband and life-partner. He is my rock. I try to be his.

And I especially thank my loving children and grandchildren, and so many dear friends—near and far—for your support and good will when you learned about this book project.

Finally, I offer a small hallelujah to the amazing 95-year-old couple, Gail Myers and Phyllis Dokken Ross, whose photograph graces the cover of this book.

You are all in my heart—and you may find yourselves in this book as well. Onward.

CONTENTS

ONE

OLD LOVE

*Take chances when you're young so you can
tell stories when you're old.*

—www.livelifehappy.com

My Mother's . . . Day
The Sock Tree
Sexy Aging
Woodchucks
LoveU2
Clown School
Affective Affirmation
Rules of Engagement
Reach Out. And Touch.
Baby Love
Young at Heart
Summer Wedding

MY MOTHER'S . . . DAY

If my mom were still alive, I would take her out to an after-church brunch today. She would be wearing that sandy-colored, linen jacket she thought camouflaged her rounded, osteoporotic back. There would be a pastel scarf at her neck and her gray-white hair would be freshly styled. She would have carefully polished her aluminum cane with her lace-edged handkerchief. When you hugged her, there would be the hint of lavender sachet.

Her excitement about the day would be sweet and real. On Mother's Day, she was almost assured a call from each of her children and grandchildren. One of them would have arranged a corsage and she would want her picture taken wearing it, hoping to include the photo in the thank you cards she would assuredly send. They would be well-worded notes of gratitude written in delicate, flowing script, acknowledging the gift and the giver, as well as her appreciation of life in general.

In the wide, side pockets of my mother's jacket, there would be a few tissues, her church offering envelope, some mints, and probably an article from a magazine that she intended to talk with me about while we ate our brunch after church. If the subject was politics, she would have underlined the opposing views in different-colored ink to help organize the discussion she wanted us to have.

In lieu of a purse, she would have an embroidered bag that held the flattened, well-worn pillows she needed in order to sit comfortably in the hard-backed church pew. Mother would not want to linger over brunch on this particular day, desiring instead to get back to her cozy, assisted living apartment for the awaited phone calls.

She might indicate several times during the meal that she was hopeful we would play a game of Scrabble later in the day and remind me she had already laid out the board, and that she also had "some of those lemon cookies you always like."

This is the mom who grew up as the daughter of a North Dakota prairie-preacher and lost her own mother in the 1917 flu epidemic when she was barely three years old. This same mother was a staff sergeant in the Women's Marine Corps during WW II and a schoolteacher in the years before the war. My long-deceased mother graduated from Mayville State Teacher's College in North Dakota at a time when most women did not go to college, let alone graduate, and she had her first child when she was in her thirties . . . and then had two more.

It's surprising what you remember about your mother on a day dedicated to doing just that. The mom I remember would tie a knotted arrangement of nylon stockings around her morning newspaper once she had read it and lower it over her balcony railing to share with the person in the apartment below. As my siblings and I were growing up, this same mother put a shower cap over the smoke alarm when she baked so it wouldn't "act up." She preferred her children not act up either, but she never admonished them with a scolding, but rather by quietly reciting the Golden Rule.

Remember this rule. And remember to tell your stories—your own mother's stories and your family stories as well. Make them memorable.

THE SOCK TREE

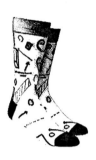

My husband gave me a "sock tree" for my birthday. I think the idea came from an early morning conversation weeks before. We were readying ourselves for the day and I noted the weather had become cooler and warmer clothing might be necessary. I happened to mention, "I have absolutely no socks to wear". . . or something to that effect.

It amazes me what husbands sometimes hear and don't hear. I know I've made other early morning comments more memorable than that one; those would be comments that resulted in complete inaction. Like the time I said, "I think we should start planning a vacation to some place balmy," or all the times I've said, "I think we need to replace the stove." This would be the stove that's as old as the house we live in, the one whose oven temperature fluctuates 10 – 15 degrees below what the dial reads. Yes, that stove.

But, returning to the subject at hand. The result of our exchange this particular morning was a birthday present like no other. It was a tall and lovely glass vase in which several dozen hangers had been reworked into wire stems with little hooks at the end (I'd been wondering about our dwindling supply of coat hangers).

On each metal hook hung a pair of patterned socks festooned with curly ribbons, and hanging among the socks and ribbons there was a variety of birthday cards that denoted my over sixty-five status. My favorite card said, "Old people are so nice and cute and funny. I love old people."

When you opened the card, it read, "But you're my favorite one." Aw shucks.

One card made me laugh out loud. On the outside it said, "The key to a long life involves a strict exercise regimen, a low-fat, low-salt, low sugar diet, and a low alcohol intake." And inside it said, "Which explains why old people are so cranky." There was even a card from the dog suggesting, "Me? Forget your birthday? What do you think I am . . . a cat?"

There were many birthday cards. He had signed none of them, perhaps thinking we should become more focused on recycling? The hole punched in the upper left hand corner of each card near the fold might make it less than ideal. If you get a birthday card from me containing a small punch hole, take note . . . it has a history.

Each fall, denoting the passage of another year, I reflect on my life experiences. My mother called it "counting your blessings." Women my age and older who participate in "The Older Women's Project" reflect all year long (www.oldwomensproject.org). Many women say they don't discover their authentic selves until after age sixty.

This year, my husband's endearing gift made me particularly reflective. It launched me into a triple-digit count of accumulated blessings. I thought about the words of sixty-something author/activist Barbara McDonald, "I like growing old, I say to myself in surprise." I also thought about the poet, May Sarton, who in her seventies said, "I'm more of myself than I've ever been."

Yes I am. And I am blessed with a husband who keeps my feet warm and my heart happy.

SEXY AGING

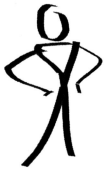 A few years ago, I was asked to speak to a group of older adult men with an average age of approximately seventy-two. The presentation they wanted me to give was on sexuality and aging. Without hesitation, I agreed. I actually agreed. Am I nuts?

Sometimes I suspect I get a little full of myself when it comes to aging issues, and I think I can write or talk about anything. In this situation, however, it's not hubris (that "too full of oneself" attitude). At least I don't think so. I happen to have information on this topic, worth-talking-about information.

I had recently attended a lecture on sexuality and aging (the term "lecture" seems at odds with the topic, don't you think?) The presentation was titled "Seniors and Sexuality: Experiencing Intimacy in Later Life." The presenter was a sixty-something woman, who was portly and fairly severe-appearing at first glance. She seemed an unlikely presenter on a subject of this kind, but she knew her stuff and now I know her stuff.

She said that the best sex was much more about intimacy than sexuality. Intimacy is made up of five things: mutuality, a sense of caring, shared values and goals, physical encounters, and commitments.

Many illustrations were used to portray sexual relationships. Most of them seemed bliss-filled and complex, and it's always better if the five-part intimacy model is firmly in place. It's clear to me that as we get older it becomes more complicated. The issues range from disease conditions that inhibit or deter two people from physical or emotional closeness to medications that have mutuality-reducing side effects. Other things can interfere, too, such as loyalty to a deceased spouse, competence (perceived or real), or concerns about body image.

I want to explore more fully the whole idea that sex has healing power. There's good solid research to support this statement. The facts state that married folks (1) live longer and (2) experience less depressive illness. The question becomes "Is this because of more frequent sexual experiences, simple companionship, or some aspect of personality that's linked to being married?" A Scottish study tried to figure it out and found (bingo) it was the sex. It was a large research project, too—including 3,500 men. Researchers found a strong link between regular sexual relations and length of life. I looked for a similar study focused on women. I'm still looking.

There is research to show that "a good sexual encounter has a positive effect on almost every part of your body . . . brain, heart, and immune system." One European study in the 1980s found that people who reported having sexual relations twice a week experienced half as many heart attacks over a ten-year time period. There's also a particularly intriguing examination of how regular intimacy boosts the immune system and helps fight off colds and other infections.

I pulled from lots of solid, science-based information for my presentation. That was my strategy: use the science, tell a few stories . . . and use no personal examples.

WOODCHUCKS

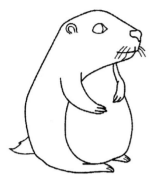

I have given up—I'm succumbing. All week there's been a phase I cannot get out of my mind. It's totally distracting. I fall asleep with it, and when I wake up it's still running through my head. Unless I cleanse it from my thinking soon, I might go slightly mad.

Here's the phrase: "How much wood would a woodchuck chuck if a woodchuck could chuck wood?" Say it a few times fast and it makes you a little dizzy. What exactly is a woodchuck anyway? How do you "chuck" wood? I mean, really, you "chop" wood and "stack" wood, and the best thing to do with wood (besides building houses and high-quality breadboards) is to burn it in your fireplace on a rainy day while reading a good book and drinking a cup of hot chocolate. Now there's a vision I would really love to have running constantly through my head.

But let's get back to the issue at hand. In case something of this nature is distracting you, I'd like to share how I'm choosing to tackle this problem. My first idea is to look up the word "woodchuck" using the Internet. But as I start to do this, I find myself reflecting, *Just how would I deal with this problem without the Internet?*

At this exact moment, our home Internet system becomes nonfunctional. There are error messages galore. I reboot. It comes back up, but then it gets constipated. Stuck—nothing moves. I reboot again and there's still no access. The word "woodchuck" must have done it. It's probably a code word of some kind. Oops, spoke too soon. Our system is now back up and running.

Oh. My. Gosh. A woodchuck is actually a groundhog; in some areas of the country, it's called a "land-beaver." No wonder I am thinking about this so intently. I have a work history on the faculty at a university that has a beaver as its mascot. There must be some sort of undone work-related activity I am subliminally channeling.

As I read on, using the always-interesting but sometimes not entirely accurate www.wikipedia.org, I'm reminded that "woodchuck-beavers" (my phrase, not theirs) are quite canny creatures. In addition to weather forecasting, they're frequently involved in medical research on liver cancer. There's loads of interesting information to absorb, including the fact these not-so-little mammals are members of the rodent family. This, by the way, is not a vision I choose to explore further.

I think this approach is working for me because the more information I have, the better I feel. Let's move on to an improved understanding of the word "chucking." The *Oxford English Dictionary* indicates it has multiple definitions including "to toss" or "to throw." But my favorite description of "chuck" is "to squeeze fondly or playfully, especially under the chin."

At this moment, my husband enters the room, sees me huddled over my computer, and asks, "So . . . what's the topic this time?" And I say, "I'm writing about woodchucks."

Quick wit that he is, my spouse responds with, "Any recipes involved?" And then he chucks me tenderly under the chin. Honest—he really did. Talk about distracting.

LOVEU2

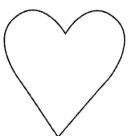

Here's the scene. My daughter is visiting for the week-end and we're driving in the countryside, off on a small adventure. I'm at the wheel. I've not spent much time with her recently and we're reconnecting.

Jen's multi-tasking. She's talking to me, checking messages on her phone, and setting up my cell phone with numbers I call frequently. (And yes, it's true; I've had that phone for over a year and have not established a call list.) I'm aware that one minute of button pushing by my daughter will save me countless hours over the next few months. I suspect she is too.

Suddenly my lovely (helpful) daughter exclaims (actually she sort of shouts) "Omigosh, mom! You have seventeen text messages!" I'm thinking, *Is that a good thing?* Apparently I've been receiving typed (text) messages on my phone for months without realizing it. She scrolls through them. Many are from her. All those times I thought she should be keeping in better touch, she actually was.

Keeping my eyes on the road, I hear her say, "I'm going to text you right now." (She really means "test.")

I tell her I'll retrieve the message when we reach our destination. I need to focus on the route. I've lost sight of my usual set of geographic markers and I'm not sure we're on the right road. I say this out loud. I think Jen rolls her eyes (just a bit) while she turns her phone into a keyboard and types. Seconds later, my phone lets out an unfamiliar "bong."

It bongs again just as we round the corner and see our destination. I look at my cell phone screen. The message reads, "We R so LOST." I think, *No, we aren't dear daughter. We are, in fact, finding ourselves—in new ways on uncharted turf.*

I love having adult children. I relish the fact that they know how to do things I don't. I cherish their breezy ways and their spontaneous energy. These same children who were such challenges in their teens and early twenties have finally come of age. Whoever said, "You do not know who your child has actually become until he/she gets to be age twenty-eight?" I cannot attribute this quote to anyone specific, and I'm thinking perhaps I made it up—but then I do have three children and lots of remembered angst.

None today—angst that is. Today we are involved in such things as choosing and purchasing garden plants in out-of-the-way places. We spent the morning culling through dusty storage boxes and then had a slightly decadent lunch that included lots of laughter.

When Jen was younger, I remember reading a book by psychologist-turned-author Mary Pipher. The book, *Reviving Ophelia*, warned mothers about the many challenges their teenage daughters face. There was a special caution about "electronic communities." I look over at my technologically savvy, cell phone-competent, happy-and-independent daughter and feel only pride.

I text Jenna, just to be sure I've got the newly-acquired skill down. "UR wonderful" is what I tell her. Her response is "UR2." Then I remember another Mary Pipher quote, "It's in the shelter of each other that people live."

CLOWN SCHOOL

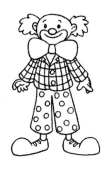

My husband tells me I have no sense of humor. Well, he did say it once, quite emphatically as I recall. It was in response to my frowning at an amusing but somewhat sarcastic joke. To me, sarcasm is sharp and biting. I like soft, safe humor. I lean toward personal stories, especially those that are true or partially true and heavy on embellishments. The extravagant exaggeration in the "Ole and Lena" jokes comes to mind. "Ole wore both of his winter jackets when he painted his house last week. The directions on the can said, 'Put on two coats.'"

I will admit my sense of humor needs work. I often forget the punch line to a joke, but once I remember it and am able to offer up the entire funny anecdote, I feel the need to explain the joke—which is one of the least funny things you can do. Someone told me this tendency can be cultural, and that being spontaneously funny is harder for Norwegians because we tend to over-analyze situations. You think? Uff-dah.

My spouse's sense of humor is fully developed. He has an undeniably quick wit and uses topical humor brilliantly. Our son-in-law recently had a corner-turning birthday and we sent him a card containing a monetary gift. He thanked us in a text message saying it took him a week to open the card because he was in denial. My hubby quickly responded with, "Are you kidding? I have shoes older than you."

This is the same husband who once suggested we go to Clown School after we retired so we could entertain at children's parties. But then we retired, and as a result we were more available to attend our own grandchildren's birthday parties. We saw the post-birthday cake pandemonium at these parties and mutually agreed that two people in their seventh decade cavorting around in costumes in front of a dozen three-year-olds was definitely not a good idea. Besides, we were flummoxed about how our hearing aids would function when tucked under a Clarabelle Clown wig—and those big floppy feet you have to wear are a definite fall hazard.

Humor is tricky, and apparently it changes as we age. A 2014 article in *The Atlantic* summed it up well. In it, the author suggested that abrasive or hard-nosed humor is not received well by older adults. The findings were drawn from a study discussed in the *Journal of Psychology and Aging*, which found that older adults do not like "aggressive" humor. They like "affiliative" humor that's loaded with "jokes that bring people together through a funny or awkward situation."

One example given in the study is the Golden Girls episode in which the women try to buy condoms and suffer an embarrassing price check. I remember that episode. I will not try to restate it in detail here and explain why it's funny. But I might try to find some old Golden Girls videos and get my hubby to join me in front of the television for an evening of laughter-filled viewing. I will provide the slightly buttered popcorn and he can be counted on to offer clever quips to enhance the experience. Yah sure, you betcha.

AFFECTIVE AFFIRMATION

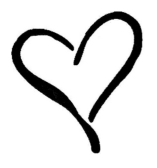

Over the course of our marriage, my husband and I have had a running discussion about marital affirmation. I do not see him offering up enough of the encouraging comments that women need to hear—at least not what this woman needs. He is very good at many things, but not that. Maybe I just require more affirmation than the average wife of multiple decades. I googled "women's need for affirmation" and was overwhelmed with articles about "the power of praise and encouragement" Anyone who has toilet trained a two-year-old knows this—but we might not apply it in marriage as much as we do in parenting.

There was a *Wall Street Journal* article published a few years ago; I think the piece was titled something like, "Want Great Marriage Advice? Ask a Divorced Person." In the article, psychologist and researcher Terri Orbuch, from the University of Michigan's Institute for Social Research, identified the importance of "being more positive" about and toward the person you're married to. She called it "affective affirmation."

"Affective affirmation" has four components (Are you listening dear?) The first is "How often does your spouse show love?" Examples include spontaneous for-no-reason-at-all hugs and frequent hand-holding. The second is "How often does your spouse make you feel good about the kind of person you are?" I have a great example of this. When I overhear my husband talking to someone in a social setting and he doesn't know I'm listening, and he mentions me with pride or praise, I feel very tender toward him. Sometimes the feeling lasts for days. (I know I have never mentioned this to him.)

The third component in affective affirmation is "How often does your spouse make you feel good about having your own ideas and ways of doing things?" This one surprised me. I'm not sure I do this well at all, and perhaps I need to work on it. My husband does it magnificently. (I don't think I ever told him this either.) Apparently, it's a quite pivotal issue for men. By the way, this particular body of research concluded that men need "affective affirmation" more than women. Who knew? Apparently, both men and women are not particularly informed about affirmation overall and often get stuck on "maintenance communication." Research suggests that once this happens, marital satisfaction can start sliding downhill.

There is one final component. The Orbuch study concluded that couples were happier and felt more affirmed if their spouses frequently made life interesting or exciting by doing something out of the ordinary. For example, my husband bought me a solar system for my birthday. Actually, he got me a loving birthday card and I bought a huge mobile of the solar system myself. Then he hung the "planetary monstrosity" (his exact words) from the ceiling in my home study while I was gone—all by himself. It required two hours and a ten-foot ladder. And the directions were in German. He did this for me and it looks absolutely amazing. As affirmations go, it was "over the moon."

RULES OF ENGAGEMENT

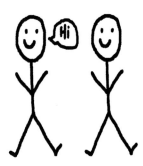

I have a beautiful young friend who got married recently, and I dedicate what I am about to write to this just-pledged couple. I offer them "rules of engagement."

Let me set the stage. It's a story I've told many times. My husband and I have been married for over thirty years. It's been good—sometimes exquisitely so. It was the second marriage for both of us and, not surprisingly, there have been hurdles. We brought together three not-very-willing children and my daughter's highly irritable cat, and set out on a trek across four states to set up a common household, taking with us an ice cooler full of cheesecake, wedding leftovers.

It was our blended family's cross-country "honeymoon." Two days into it, I was driving an aging sedan and my brand-new husband was responsible for a jam-packed U-Haul and two preteen girls. On this particular day, the yowling cat (in a padded carrier, fortunately) and my ten-year-old stepson were sitting on the seat next to me.

As I recall, it all began with an innocent discussion about political candidates, prompted by something provocative on the car radio. I'd been looking for anything to conversationally capture this young boy's attention and this seemed to do it. Not surprisingly, he shared his father's political orientation—which has changed since then, but at that time it was vastly different from my own.

Tiny alarm bells went off as my new son and I continued chatting. As many premarital challenges as we had surmounted, and as many obstacles as we would assuredly face with our newly con-structed family, this business of political differences seemed to have the greatest potential to unsettle me. I was definitely not being my "best self." What is it about "things political" that has to be so polarizing?

Our caravan stopped for lunch and we maintained an on-going discussion about a certain candidate's proclivities and the high-drama approaches of a select few running for office. (Do keep in mind, this was thirty years ago!). At first, I elected to think of the discussion as educational, but then less so. It seemed to be turning into a "girls against guys" sort of dialogue, as my stepdaughter put it. At this point, I'm thinking, *Uh-oh, this is not the way to launch a lifetime of familial bliss.*

Our third night on the road, we decided to establish "rules of engagement" about future exchanges and our communication in general. Over the decades, we have faithfully observed these "ground rules" in potentially divisive situations. They are very simple:

1. No cheap shots
2. Issues, not personalities
3. Anyone can "call time" at any point in a discussion and regroup to reconsider their position

Our familial exchanges have continued to incorporate these rules and the discussions are still lively, especially when any of our smart, feisty grandchildren are at the table and involved in the dialogue.

As I continue learning over the decades, this is what I have come to know about marriage and family life—and about the world in general. We are better at talking about our differences in thoughtful, solution-oriented ways when we have a few basic rules of engagement. It is then we are more likely to become our collective "best selves."

REACH OUT. AND TOUCH.

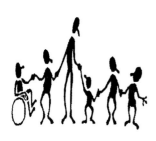 Find somebody to love. This might sound like a directive, but consider it an invitation. It's actually a 1960s song, originally recorded by the rock group Jefferson Airplane. It has been described as a song that "implores us to find love that will nurture and protect us through the tough times."

Maybe you will remember it better if I share more of the lyrics:

Don't you want somebody to love?
Don't you need somebody to love?
Wouldn't you love somebody to love?

The last line is actually the best:

You better find somebody to love.

When sung with musical fervor, it really does sound like a directive to take action. And so you must, especially if you're nearing a holiday.

Let me explain. My thoughts come after reading an on-line blog sent to me by several different people. The "rant" starts out, "Christmas is a cheery season" and the blog acknowledges the layers of published festivities and greenery-filled holiday happenings. But then it singles out "sleigh bell imagery, excessive decorations, and shopping discounts." The blog suggests that "self-identifying Christians," who should be the purveyors of the very best Christmas thinking, are trending down in numbers. It states, without equivocation, that the author—Laurie Ortov, whom I do not know but admire because she writes boldly— believes Christmas has largely become "a springboard for irrational spending . . . and financial hangovers."

This takes me back to my earlier invitation/directive. Find somebody to love. You have the opportunity to alter the splashy retail emphasis of any pending holiday and reach out in a way you might not have considered previously. If you are of a religious bent, you might do it more naturally. But, maybe not. Anyone can search and find. Again, let me explain.

For older adults, the holidays are often about loneliness, not comfort and joy. Ponder these facts. Nearly half of women over age seventy-five live alone. In some areas of the country, it's well over half. And reportedly almost half of all grandparents live more than 200 miles from at least one grandchild. Here is an even more sobering fact: many elders are estranged from any children or grandchildren they do have. Many aging women and men have no family to call upon— none. The potential for loneliness and isolation throughout the entire year is enormous, but during the holiday season it's sadly even more overwhelming. So it is up to all us to change this alarming situation.

"Finding somebody to love" can happen because of a telephone call you haven't made before. Maybe it's just the beginning, and you set up a reliable series of weekly calls. Maybe it's through offering a random and unexpected hug during a grocery store encounter, and then you offer to go to the store for your aging neighbor on a regular basis.

Loving someone means providing a listening ear, a small gift, or a commitment to on-going conversation. There are organizations that help lonely elders, but you're probably better at this kind of outreach than they are. You know it's important. You got this—right?

BABY LOVE

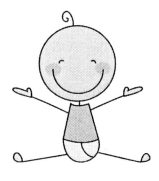

Indulge me as I reflect on the birth of a most remarkable baby. All babies are, of course, but this one happens to be mine. Well, sort of. I intend to write oh-so-tenderly about my youngest grandson. Maybe what I'm going to say about babies and the birthing process will call up memories of happy-endings or new beginnings in your own life.

He was "a miracle baby" according to the doctors who delivered him. In a moment of exhausted jubilation following a lengthy emergency caesarean delivery on New Year's Eve five years ago, the surgeon said, "It is amazing this baby was ever conceived, let alone successfully carried for thirty-three weeks." He was lodged deep under the forty-year-old mother's rib cage and the first-time mom, my daughter, had a severe case of preeclampsia (high blood pressure and related conditions not favorable to an easy birth).

But as happens with miracles, it all went well and this youngest addition to our family entered the world. He was named Jordan Kaleo Kai (his middle name means "voice of the ocean"). When he was born he weighed 3 lbs. 4 oz. "Less than some of the cans of soup in our pantry" is how my husband put it. But Jordan gained ten grams the first day and breathed on his own the second day. Everyone in the family believed he grinned just a little when he heard his name. Early on, you could see his personality and know he was going to be a rascal.

"Jordan boy," his loving parents called softly to him, as they stood outside his isolate in a Portland-based neonatal intensive care unit. His heart rate monitor bumped up at the sound of their voices. After the first day, first mom, and then dad, was allowed to hold him "skin-to-skin." As they held him, you could hear the soft hum of Hawaiian music (dad is a Maui boy) or the coo of the "By-oh" song, a wordless tune I invented long ago when my daughter was an infant.

Jordan entered the world with an APGAR of 7 and 9. These are really good scores considering the trauma he went through during the birthing process. Ever heard of this? The APGAR is the very first test given to a newborn to quickly evaluate physical condition at one minute and five minutes after birth. It seems like it might have some relevance to older adults, too. (I will need to ponder this concept in a later chapter of this book.)

The letters in APGAR stand for:

1. Appearance (skin coloration)
2. Pulse (heart rate)
3. Grimace (reflex irritability i.e. if stimulated, does he respond)
4. Activity (movement and muscle tone), and
5. Respiration (breathing rate and effort).

Health professionals subjectively score each category in a 0 – 2 range at one minute and five minutes after birth and total the scores on a 1 – 10 scale. It's rare for any newborn to get a 10.

This remarkable little guy wowed everyone in the delivery room, and every year of his life since his birth he has continued to amaze and engage our family. On almost any scale, he would be considered a definite "ten." Ah yes, I know. I am biased as well as smitten. Love that feeling.

YOUNG AT HEART

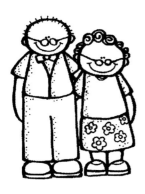

Many years ago, an eleven-year-old classmate gave me a box of multi-flavored lifesavers as a Valentine gift. My parents thought I was far too young to be getting gifts from boys, but following a family discussion I was allowed to keep the present. My sister and I sucked on those colorful little discs for weeks. And that earnest fifth grader who offered up the gift, well . . . he will remain in my heart forever.

I was reminded of those lifesavers while going through my deceased aunt's estate, which included a multitude of musty boxes filled with remembrances from her youth. There were long-saved, chocolate wrappers and several corsages pressed inside the pages of a small book. There was a hatbox full of porcelain-headed dolls and dozens of photograph albums, one displaying a happy twenty-something woman wearing a sundress with a halter-top. She looked young at heart. Another photo, nearby in the album, showed my aunt seventy some years later with spectacles and wrinkles, but I thought she looked young at heart there, too.

I'm in a thoughtful, remembering mood. Reflect with me, if you will. I have a few important questions. Let's start with this one: How old do I look? (There's a photograph in the back of this book, so you can easily decide.) How about you? How old do you look? If there's a mirror nearby, glance into it. It's not just about looks, though. How old do you feel?

I like to think I look younger than my seventy-one years. I definitely *feel* younger, and no matter how you answered my question about how old I look, *it's more important how I answered it*. People with the best sense of personal well-being feel younger than they are. I believe my aunt, who was energetic and youthful-appearing into her nineties, only started *being* old in the last year or two of her life—when she started *feeling* old.

A Brandeis University study done by psychologist Margie Lachman found that people with the greatest sense of well-being feel younger than they actually are, no matter what others might think regarding their age.

The study was designed so that participants looked at photographs of one another and estimated age. Before age forty, the task was easier. It seems there was greater accuracy in targeting the age of the person pictured. After age forty, a large percentage (58 – 61 percent) did not think the people in the pictures looked as old as their actual age. But some thought they looked even older (22 – 24 percent). No matter what the outside assessment, the most important finding was that other people's conclusions had little relevance. Your opinion of yourself was found to be the most important in terms of personal contentment.

How old you feel is linked to your sense of well-being. The study found that believing you look your age or younger, but not too much younger than others think you are, is self-protective.

Today I'm feeling about fifty-nine, and despite the death and disability of friends and loved ones, a family estrangement, and a few irksome aches and pains, I'm contented with my life, young at heart, even.

Perhaps most importantly, I have every intention of continuing to feel that way through the ages.

SUMMER WEDDING

In the off chance you have a summer wedding on your calendar, I'm offering a few ideas to encourage full enjoyment of the occasion. Think of this as a tip sheet of sorts. "Five Rules for Aging Adults Attending a Summer Wedding." After all, we might need a little refresher about what we originally committed to, or a new perspective on sustaining the magic of married love.

I've researched wedding etiquette, and there seems an abundance of things you're NOT supposed to do at a wedding. However, I'm choosing to focus on the positive things aging guests (all guests, for that matter) can do to make any wedding sweeter and more memorable.

My husband and I had two weddings scheduled during a recent summer. The first nuptials involved a patio celebration for my thirty-something niece. The bride and groom are extraordinary in many ways, and both of them sport extensive tattoos, full arm and partial neck designs. Their tattoos were nicely on display, with the bride's strapless dress and the groom in his short sleeves and colorful canvas sneakers. Many of the guests had tattoos as well. First Rule: Stay open to the increasing informality of the wedding dress code. Do not stare at the tattoos. By the way, wear your dancing shoes.

Second Rule: Bring stories, fun and funny tales about the bride and groom—the kind of silly-friend and family stories they haven't heard before or maybe they have and the couple would like the world to know. Make it your goal—if you get a chance to tell your story in front of the guests—to do it in a way that makes the newly married couple look at each other with misty acknowledgement. If the bridal party has too much going on to listen to the stories you came prepared to share, use them as icebreakers with the other guests, whose names and histories you probably should know—but do not. That's okay. No rules there.

Here's a story. My niece, the bride, has a four-year-old daughter from her previous marriage. Little Adeline was the active center of the small wedding party. When asked if she had a story to share, she catapulted into her mother's arms, tiny little hands on each side of her mom's face, and looking directly into her mother's eyes, she said, "My mommy is very beautiful." Then she turned to the assembly of enchanted guests and said, "And, if you will all be happy, you will be beautiful, too."

This is a true story, and it is also Rule Three. Make all the stories you tell true and positive, and short. (Rule Four.)

Rule Five is a bit more complex. It involves the Japanese word "aikido," which is a style of communication that encourages aligning yourself with the energy of the person you are talking with, i.e., put yourself in that person's place and lean into what they are saying. Communication can get a little complex when family members have not seen one another for a while or new family clans are being formed—especially if there's a lot of champagne involved.

Make a special effort to practice aikido, on and off the dance floor. If you can pull that off, you will almost assuredly be happy and beautiful.

TWO

FRIENDLIER AGING

*How old would you be if you didn't know
how old you was?*
—Satchel Paige

Don't Let Me Call You Sweetheart
Cousins Counted
Old and Funny
That Would Be Lightbulb
Whimsy
Avocados on Tuesday
Gotcha
Stop Acting Old
Forgetting Older
Praiseworthy
Reach Out. Lift Up.

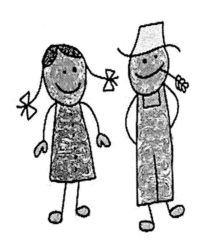

DON'T LET ME CALL YOU SWEETHEART

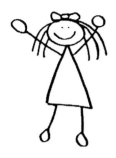 It happened again today. I was in a grocery store and queried a clerk about the location of a particular food item. She responded with, "It's on the next aisle, left-hand side, sweetie." As I rolled my cart in that direction, she called after me, "Have a good day, hon."

Earlier in the week at another retail establishment, I was addressed as "sweetie-pie" and "honey-bun." I am frequently called "my dear" and "dearie." A few weeks ago, I was referred to as "Missy." I am over seventy years old, so what were they thinking?

Is it just me? Does anyone else find this type of sugary terminology a little demeaning? Before I go into a rant about how older people might like to be addressed, I want to put something on the record. I totally understand the folks who use these terms of endearment are well-intentioned. And I know some of my age peers often smile graciously when referred to in a similar way. Some people actually like it very much. Not me.

I do have an exception. If my spouse were to call me "sweetheart," I would be momentarily enchanted as well as very surprised. I think he called me "honey" once a few years ago, and there is the occasional "dear." But if he were to call me "honey-bun," I would start to be concerned about his possible cognitive loss.

People who study communication have told me that the most polite way of addressing an older woman you do not know is "Ma'am," which is short for "Madame." I rather like the idea of being called "Madame" by people I don't know or by new acquaintances. I'm less sure about that other term, "Ma'am," but I prefer it to "Missy." This all seems easier for men. They can be called "Sir" at any age and it's viewed as a term of respect.

In the press, people in their retirement years are usually referred to as "seniors" or "senior citizens," although the latter term is reported to be "annoying to just about everyone." When politicians say "our" seniors, it seems particularly patronizing. I have seen the term "older Americans" used more often lately, and the people I talk to sometimes resonate with it. The academic press defends the use of the terminology "older adult" or "elder" as being "more respectful." I recently read an article that used the term "super adult" and I sort of grimaced. I also know some literature on aging has introduced the term "gero-ager," but I cannot imagine it will catch on.

A column in the *New York Times* years ago reported that when asked about the best terminology to use for people over age sixty-five, the president of "Generational Targeted Marketing" said, "For heavens' sake, don't call them anything. Instead refer to 'stage of life' and lifestyle. People in the baby boomer generation really do not like to be reminded of the fact they are no longer young."

I am fine with the fact I am no longer young. "Delightfully old" is how I like to think about myself. In response to this self-affirmation, my teenage granddaughter would probably say, "Sweet."

COUSINS COUNTED

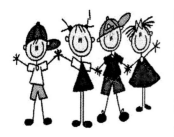

Here's a question you're probably not asked very often. How many cousins do you have? Reflect for a minute. Do a quick count.

I have nineteen cousins. Two of them showed up on our doorstep recently. They were Norwegian-speaking men in their later decades and they told stories I'd never heard and recalled events I'd long forgotten. They provided elaboration on their lives—and I gained insight into my own.

The visit prompted thoughts about the role cousins might play as we age. They are, after all, our age peers—once removed from siblings. We share common ancestors and so they offer an indisputable link to our genetic core. Powerful stuff if you let it loose. Why have I not thought about this before? It might be the way to increase social connections for aging adults who don't have enough friends. It's a particularly important issue, because as we age we are at substantial risk of losing affiliations—just when we need them the most.

My husband seemed to enjoy the unexpected visit from the lovely Norwegians, so I posed the idea of a road trip during which we would visit all our respective cousins and catalogue the experience. This was not well-received. I knew the minute he raised one eyebrow and looked at me like I'd lost my mind that we would probably not be going. But my spouse (who has even more cousins that I do) is willing to keep talking about cousinship. I'm waiting for just the right moment to re-spring the trip idea.

Once you start considering this topic, it's hard to put it aside until you've mentally gathered up all the children of your various aunts and uncles and accounted for them. The process itself has many benefits. It can serve as excellent cognitive stimulation and might even help improve your memory. Really—I'm serious. This could replace cross-word puzzles and Sudoku.

Don't forget to categorize your cousins. Deceased and non-deceased is fairly easy, but the breakdown of first, second, and third cousins, and the interplay of half-cousins and step-cousins can be a bit more challenging. Once you have the total, the possible social interactions are huge. Cousin relationships offer an intergenerational opportunity we have definitely not been maximizing. Just thinking about it makes me want to write a letter to one of my cousins telling him (or her) how my week is going.

One caveat, if you don't have a lot of cousins, maybe you could borrow somebody else's. I have a cousin near Fargo, North Dakota who would be delighted to be contacted—as long as I vouched for you and you liked lefse.

There's a lot to ponder. And I have a trip to plan.

OLD AND FUNNY

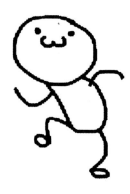

It's been reported that children laugh 300 – 400 times a day and adults laugh only an average of seventeen. Not good. But hear this. I randomly asked a dozen or so older adults how often they laughed each day and nobody said seventeen. They used far smaller numbers. Take a moment and do a self-check. What's your average? Why not use yesterday as your baseline.

We need more laughter in our lives because laughing promotes an undisputed sense of overall well-being. Think of it as an internal massage or a brief but rejuvenating aerobic work-out. Research (University of Maryland, Vanderbilt University) tells us laughing positively affects blood pressure, increases immune system strength, and helps manage pain. Granted, these are often small studies and design flaws are sometimes present. Possibly there's also a little researcher bias. After all, who wants to discover laughing is NOT good for you.

Maybe more laughter on a daily basis is too much to ask. Maybe we should just go for more smiling behavior. Did you know there are two kinds of smiles? There's the authentic "Duchenne Smile," originally identified by Guillaume Duchenne, a researcher-neurologist. This kind of smile is when people get all crinkled up in their forehead and nose-eye area with one of those radiant, "light up your life" smiles. Then there's the other kind of smile, the "Pan American Smile." This is the polite, courteous, "professional smile."

Now that we're smiling, I have information to share about a larger research study. Apparently psychologists at the University of California, Berkeley did a longitudinal study that used high school yearbook photos. They assessed over 140 photographs to determine which person had a "Duchenne" smile and which had a "Pan American" smile. (They eliminated photographs of non-smiling graduates.)

It was about half and half in terms of how many individuals had each kind of smile. But then it got interesting. The researchers followed up and re-contacted the women (yes, they were all women) when they were 27, 43, and 52 years of age, in order to determine their level of happiness and life satisfaction. What do you think they found? The Duchenne smiles won, hands down. They were more likely to be happily married and their overall level of life-satisfaction was higher. (I wish they'd asked how many times the women laughed each day.)

This brings me back to laughing. Did you know dogs laugh? I really think they do. The playful, open-mouthed sound they make when they're running to catch a ball or mouthing a soft toy is the dog's way of "laughing." I'm not sure if there's any real research to support this, but I read about an experiment that used the recorded sounds of dogs laughing. It was played over the loudspeaker in an animal shelter. The sound came on and the dogs ceased their barking. Yes, they did. I won't suggest they all started laughing, but they did quit barking.

This is potentially powerful stuff. Remember the earlier estimate you made about the number of times you laugh in a given day. Bump it up.

THAT WOULD BE LIGHTBULB

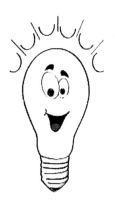

Has this ever happened to you? Let's say you're responding to a friend's email message and you become very excited about what she's suggesting. You rush to acknowledge her invitation, typing fast and hastily pushing "send." Moments later you feel strangely unsettled about the reply you sent. So you retrieve your email from the "sent" file and you're absolutely flabbergasted by the words you put together, or you're embarrassed. Maybe you're very embarrassed.

Recently I received an email query from a friend and I wanted to be quickly affirming. But instead of saying, "That would be delightful," I typed, "That would be lightbulb." I did not even realize I had offered up that phrase until my friend came back with a positive comment about the term. I think it made her smile. It made me smile, and as a result all week long my husband and I have been saying, "That would be lightbulb" when anything really interesting, creative, or special comes our way. We've had rather dark and dreary weather, so this phrase has helped us get through it.

Now, maybe you're thinking, *I do not make these kinds of mistakes. I'm a pen and paper person who uses envelopes with commemorative stamps.* This is totally fine—there's less chance of misinterpretation. Although when I was a freshman in college, I did mail a letter to a young man with whom I was totally smitten in an envelope addressed to my parents. Now that was really awkward.

But let's stay in the present. If email mishaps are the type of problem you and I share, you might already know that texting can be an even bigger issue because the autocorrect function in text messaging is ridiculously overzealous. The website www.damnyouautocorrect.com discusses how using the word "mistress" when you meant to say "mattress," and then stringing the words together in yet another autocorrected text (after you've realized what's happening) can get you in a whole lot of trouble. Note to self: Do not try to over-correct the autocorrect. Smile. Laugh. Move on.

For some time, the *Huffington Post* has run a list of the funniest autocorrect exchanges that occurred over the preceding year. I just went through a recent year's list trying to find something I could use as an illustration to make you smile or laugh a little. But they are all a bit on the salty side and I am uneasy about including them here. That said, I was doubled over laughing with tears streaming down my cheeks after this little exercise.

A final and personal example: I once sent a text to my daughter-in-law right after I'd learned how to add those little colorful graphics to a text message. I am told they're called "emoticons." I thought I was offering up a heart-shape as an emoticon but I was, in fact, sending a series of texts where each message ended with a tiny picture of a toilet. Now why would you even want to have a tiny picture of a toilet as an option? I was mortified, but those messages made her laugh and I laughed, too. In fact, it seemed to improve our overall relationship enormously—as laughter often does. That would be lightbulb.

WHIMSY

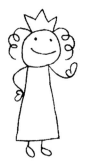 How has your week been? My week has not gone well. There was the nearly one-thousand-dollar car repair, and then my home computer lost its power supply. This was on Monday. By mid-week, my phone had started asking me for a password that I did not have—and did not know how to get—before it would allow me to retrieve any voice mail messages. Frustrating! Perhaps the problem was related to the fact that I'd dropped my phone on a hard surface earlier that same day—twice.

There was a really stinky issue involving my forgetting to remove a large bunch of freshly-picked scallions that I had purchased at a farmer's market from an airtight enclosure. The enclosure, specifically, would be the same car that had just been repaired. It's also the car that keeps indicating a tire pressure problem when there isn't one. An irksome, yellow exclamation point comes on the dashboard and I'm required to take the car back to the mechanic to have a button reset. It happens every time I have my car repaired and it makes me really cranky.

I could go on, but you get the picture. Maybe you've had a tough week, too. I concluded my karma was off tilt or the barometer was falling. Maybe I needed more sleep—or less coffee.

Then I saw the phrase "I am fairly certain that given a cape and a nice tiara, I could save the world." I saw this in a store window on a piece of cardboard artwork when I was walking the dog early one morning. It made me smile and even laugh a little. I completely forget all my other issues and difficulties for a few minutes. Isn't it amazing what calms and relaxes a person?

Not that I see myself as saving the world, but I love the fact that it might be possible. I love unexpected, slightly absurd humor that has a bit of embedded whimsy. I need to be reminded that I don't have to take life quite so seriously.

Later that same day, I bought the artwork. I'm glancing at it as I write this. The colorful design has actually sustained me over the last few days and I want to give credit to the creator—a young, happy-faced woman, whose website is www.curlygirldesign.com.

One year her company received a "LOUIE Award" for designing "the best Mother's Day card under $3.50." Apparently it used the phrase "Even if she weren't my mom . . . ." This creative little organization (their website is incredible) had two other finalists in the same contest that year. In the "Romance" category, their phrase was "I would rather do nothing with you . . ." and in the "Holiday" category it was "Mitten on every hand . . . ."

On the back of the calming piece of craft-art I purchased, there is another whimsical truism that made me smile. Be assured I will share it. Just give me another paragraph.

I have an additional point to make first. It's my personal wish for all of us as we age. Let's not get sucked down by the wear and tear of life. It would help if, maybe even just for today, no matter what our situation or circumstance, we could each find something that makes us smile—out loud.

If you're still wondering about the phrase on the back of my newly acquired art; it's "Live imperfectly with great delight."

AVOCADOS ON TUESDAYS

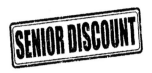

I just came back from the store. It was a simple trip for a dozen eggs, a few avocados, grated cheese, and some marmalade. As I stood ready to check out, my debit card in hand, the clerk asked me if I wanted "the senior discount."

She didn't say, "I'm not sure if you're eligible to receive our senior discount, but if you are, we do have one in effect on Tuesdays." She didn't ask if I'd heard about their "honored citizen" discount (a much preferable term, don't you think?). She didn't even smile at me.

She assumed I was over sixty-five and did the obligatory customer query before she charged me. It was Tuesday, after all. This I appreciate, of course. Although smiling at seniors seems like it should go with querying them about their discounted status. Think about that way of phrasing it for just a minute.

I have no problem looking eligible for said discount (I guess) but no matter what your age, how should you deal with this question? Here's a thought. Perhaps she had asked everyone who came through her line that day about their eligibility for a senior discount. If asked, who among us would say, "No thanks" to a reduced grocery bill? Even if you weren't sixty or older, would you say, "Can you tell me the age-cutoff for being called a senior?" Maybe you would, or maybe you would just nod—and hopefully smile a little—and take the savings.

Take the savings. There are quite a large number of discounted products and fees for older adults. No matter what our economic status, we are basically a frugal bunch in many ways and should be tuned into the possibility of cost reductions for the products we buy.

"Always ask" is my new motto. Do it before a clerk, who might have had too many chatty, slow-moving aging adults in her line already that day, asks you. It feels better to do it this way, and it puts you in control.

"Control" is a big issue as we age. We have a lot of "lost control" in our lives. We lose our vision and hearing, and jobs to retirement and spouses to death. We often feel like we lose status or visibility.

I've read that aging people in their mid-to-late sixties feel the most concern about losing control and about interactions and relationships.

But I've also read that when we get to about age seventy-five, we find our voices and our confidence rises. And it stays high and we feel very "in control." A website called www.realsimple.com and a blog titled "Five Great Things about Growing Old" might be worth looking at in this regard.

At one point it had an article about a woman named Betty Reid Soskin, who at age eighty-nine was a full-time park ranger for the Rosie the Riveter World War II National Historic Park in Richmond, California. Now there's a woman whose spirit I want to take with me when I shop for avocados on Tuesdays.

GOTCHA

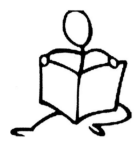 I've concluded there are certain words and phrases in the English language that are so overused they've become irksome to the ear. Communication experts and word merchants seem to agree with me. They suggest it's often phrases like "It is what it is" or "At the end of the day . . . ." May I add, "You think?"

If you're a regular reader of the *Independent Florida Alligator* (www.alligator.org) and follow their on-line blogger, Kelly Collar, you already know about "The ten most excessively used words or phrases." By the way, you're encouraged to read this blog with a light heart and an eager smile, which is a lovely way to engage. Maybe these are words that should be used more often.

There are reportedly between 150,000 and half a million words in the English language. Many experts suggest the most over-used is "awesome." In conversations I've had lately, a runner-up could be "gnarly." Did you know these two words mean almost the same thing?

Here's a bigger question. What counts as a word? These same word experts say it's impossible to be sure. Think about it like this. Is "dog" one word or two different words—a noun meaning "a kind of animal" and a verb meaning "to follow persistently"? If you make it plural, are there another two words? Is "dog-tired" a word that should be counted? What about "hot dog." One word or two? At this point, you're probably saying "Do I care?" or "Whatever . . . ." Note that both these phrases are on the "most over-used" lists, of course.

Other phrases I've heard much too frequently in recent months are "kick the can down the road" and "fiscal cliff" (some news organizations now actually ban their use). "Superfood" is definitely overused.

The website www.squidoo.com ventures into the wordsmithing realm in one article and asks the question, "When someone says 'think outside the box,' do you feel like shutting them in a box?" Are you going to scream if you hear some kid say "like, you know" one more time?"

I queried a small sample of people asking what word or phrase they felt was overused to the point of "pushing their buttons." One person said it was "the dog wants out," which I would not have put on any list of this kind, although people with dogs probably use that phrase a lot.

Several posed the word "literally." One reader told me I've used it incorrectly in the past. An article on the squidoo website helped assure that I would not do that again by suggesting "literally" is not a word to be used for emphasis. "It's a word you use when you say something should not be interpreted figuratively." For example, if you jumped so high you bumped your head, you might say, "I literally hit the ceiling." But if you were to say, "I literally worked my butt off," it doesn't mean you worked really hard. It means you don't have a butt anymore. LOL

STOP ACTING OLD

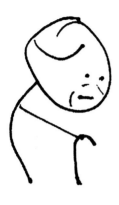

For me, it's dangerous when the checkout line at the grocery store is several people deep and I'm way in the back of the line. I stand there gazing at the "buy me" stuff positioned on either side of the aisle and then . . . I succumb. Sometimes I opt for a particularly beckoning candy item (not proud of that, but it happens), but mostly I decide to purchase a magazine . . . like I did today.

This was not just any magazine. It was billed as "the best-selling magazine for women over forty." The name suited what I was doing—adding more to my already overflowing cart and justifying it because I thought maybe I could write about the whole experience. And so I am.

What caught my eye was not just the magazine. The cover called out the various stories contained inside, including one titled "Is Sugar Aging You?" But the real eye-catcher was "How Not to Act Old." It turned out to be an excerpt from a book by the same name written by Pamela Redman Satran.

Are you ready? This could be useful. First, there was a directive about wearing a watch. It said, "A naked wrist is now as emblematic of youth as a perky butt." I'm not sure I think that's entirely true, but I might start wearing my watch less frequently and see what happens.

The article also suggested we must not (1) tell lengthy (well . . . make that "any") stories about things that happened more than eight years ago; (2) feel compelled to send birthday and thank you cards. (I thought that one was a little harsh, but it definitely lets me off the hook when I forget to send them); and (3) leave voice mail messages.

Now that last one is particularly interesting, because it has the secondary benefit of eliciting action. The author actually ran a test. She called people and did one of three things:

1. She left a lengthy message explaining an issue and requesting a return call;
2. She left a brief "call me," and (the third and most effective way in this day of caller ID);
3. She placed the call and then hung up.

As Satran summarized it, "You make them curious and they call right back." Aha! Perhaps that's at the core of not getting old at all—just keep them guessing.

Pamela's book seems to focus on eliminating actions that position aging adults less attractively with the younger generation. For example, it suggested I stop asking my teenage granddaughter questions like "How's school?" or "Are you doing something fun this summer?" I'm not sure what I should say instead, maybe something about soy lattes?

The author also advises us not to be overly cheery around teenagers. I believe this to be the default position for most adults when they feel uncomfortable about what to say to adolescents, so there's definitely work to do there—but maybe that's just me.

I'm not entirely sure about this book, but reading an excerpt definitely made me laugh—repeatedly. At the risk of seeming too cheery, that's a good thing.

FORGETTING OLDER

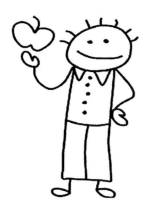

A few years ago, the following words jumped out at me from an article in *The New Yorker* written by Donald Hall, an eighty-three year-old former Poet Laureate. He quipped "If we forget for a moment we are old, we are reminded when we try to stand up . . . ."

You might recognize this statement to be true, but possibly not as engaging as I found it. Try this one. "However alert we are, and however much we think we know what will happen, antiquity remains an unknown, an unanticipated galaxy." The comments from the sage Mr. Hall are nested under the heading that reads "The View in Winter." He sees aging as "the circles growing smaller" and old age as a "ceremony of losses," but not something to be lamented. His solution to "aging well" is full immersion in fond recollection.

The same magazine, in a different article, talks about aging from a Peter Pan perspective. Think about when Peter said, "I won't grow up." The woman who has played the little imp's role on Broadway for almost two decades is Cathy Rigby, the former Olympic gymnast who looks about fourteen and is actually over sixty. She attributes successful aging to having some of Peter Pan's "sense of mischief."

It took me only twenty-one seconds at my computer to identify that there are 2,590,000 books and articles on successful aging. Quite a number of them discuss "the positivity effect," which at first sounded like something straight out of Neverland. It's usually described as a "biased tendency toward and preference for positive, emotionally gratifying experiences."

German neuroscientists found that elderly subjects who focused on life's more positive aspects had far greater emotional stability and life-contentment. Maybe they were happier because they were happy.

Lifespan theorists believe that having a positivity bias in later life means a greater emphasis on short-term rather than long-term priorities and a tendency to realistically appraise the situation but without any tendency toward negativism. I think they would suggest if we feel ourselves going down that darker path, we re-group on the spot, using humor, self-talk, or the tender advice of someone who loves us.

Let's try an illustration. This example is actually drawn from the same issue of *The New Yorker*; it was a cartoon. The drawing depicts an aging couple. The husband has a bent-head, forlorn look. His wife, who is standing close by, is saying, "But why not be happy about all the diseases you don't have?"

Toward the end of his career and well into old age himself, B.F. Skinner wrote a book about how to enjoy old age. What do you think he found to be the most important? The role and power of positivism.

Take a minute and think about the best thing that's happened to you so far today. Was it a glorious sunrise? Perhaps it was a telephone call from a dear friend, or maybe an unexpected acknowledgement.

May I suggest you gather together and store your fond recollections and pull them out whenever they are needed? Try creating a new set of "best things" tomorrow. This, and a little periodic mischief, should get you nicely through the week, and well beyond.

PRAISEWORTHY

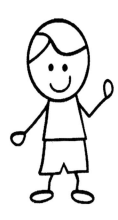

"Sandwich every bit of criticism between two thick layers of praise." This sentence might explain why Mary Kay Ash, founder of the phenomenally successful cosmetics company, did so well. It's attributed to her.

Praise can change everything. I'm not talking about compliments. This is not about "You have a beautiful smile" or "That was a great meal." These are fine statements and we need to use more of them. Research at Marquette University demonstrated that compliments are so important that even when the speaker is insincere, they are still effective. But praise is different.

A dog-eared article from a *Good Housekeeping* magazine, which I have kept for years, puts it like this: "Praise triggers the pleasure centers of the brain, producing an effect similar to antidepressants." It's "an espresso shot of confidence and good feelings." Wondrously, it also makes the person who is providing the positive comment feel good, too.

Praise glorifies. Praise begets joy. Well-delivered praise indicates we're giving our complete attention to a situation and the people involved.

It seems simple but it's not, and there are cautions. In the words of the teacher-psychologist, Haim Ginott, "Praise, like penicillin, must not be administered haphazardly." Praise is best provided in frequent small doses and best communicated one-on-one. So let's give each other praise without evaluation.

Think about the last time you acknowledged, from-the-heart, someone you care about. If it was as recently as yesterday, I salute you. If you cannot easily call up a moment in which authentic acknowledgement was given or received, I invite you to praise more.

I just finished reading Joan Dideon's *The Year of Magical Thinking*, an incredibly thoughtful book that is sobering on many levels. The author constantly remembers how many times her deceased husband said to her, "Why is it you always feel you have to be right?" It stings her in the recall. There was one incident in which she was driving the car (he was usually the driver, but age and health often change these roles). As they arrived at their destination, he commented, "Well-driven." This affirmation buoyed her and implanted itself in her memory. It might seem inconsequential in the retelling, but I resonate with it. I suspect you might, too.

I have done a little research on the nature of praise. It was launched as the result of a critical exchange my husband and I had over something that now seems trivial. In a few short minutes, we sandwiched a pot load of criticism into what could have been an informed, even pleasant, discussion. We seldom really argue, so this moment has stayed with me. Actually, it's probably the reason I am writing this. All is better now, but I learned from it.

Who hasn't had someone tell them, "If you cannot say something nice, don't say anything at all." I would amend this to reflect the positive, "If you have something nice to say, just say it." When you admire someone and you love who they are, what they do, and how they do it, tell them. Be specific.

REACH OUT. LIFT UP.

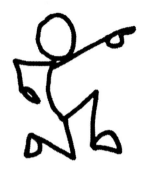

Over the last few weeks I've encountered people with enormous strength and grace. They were older rather than younger, more women than men. These individuals were dealing with life circumstances that involved debilitating illness or long-held disability. My experience was gleaned from community volunteerism. It prompted me to take a new look at resilience.

Let's define the word "resilience" as "the ability to roll with the punches. When stress, adversity, or trauma strike, you experience anger, grief, and pain, but you're able to keep functioning, physically and psychologically." Those folks at the Mayo Clinic had it pegged. They asked, "When something goes wrong, do you bounce back or fall apart?" Resilience doesn't make your problems go away, but it prompts you to harness your inner strength and look past the problems; in other words, rebound.

It's one thing to rebound if you're in a comfortable place in life with all the food and shelter you need, a bank account that gives you back-up, and caring loved ones. It is quite different if all you have is . . . you.

Let me share a few stories. I met a man recently with a history of traumatic brain injury he sustained as the result of an accident thirty years ago. He has frequent seizures and walks with what must be an agonizing lurching motion, because he can count on only one side of his body for support. He has lived independently for decades. He just turned sixty-five, and he needs a ramp to get into his house and grab bars throughout the house in order to walk around inside without falling. Perhaps you know someone like this. He has incredible resilience, but he needs a helping hand.

I met a woman in a wheelchair, who demonstrated how she precariously transfers into her non-accessible shower. This lovely elder said she had not been able to shower independently without someone watching her for over five years. She wondered if I had any ideas about modifying the shower to make it easier to use. I did, and I knew some folks who had even better ideas.

We get so caught up in our own issues that we sometimes forget the lower-income elders who have challenges that far surpass ours. Harken to this, my friends. There are plenty of opportunities to reach out—and then find you cherish the feeling that comes from offering simple support and active problem-solving.

Let me be more specific. Here is a real-world example. Make that "opportunity." As we age, many of us will live alone with chronic health conditions, and we might need a fall-alert system of some kind. It's the "I fell and I can't get up" scenario.

You know what they are, those little neck-chain pendants or wristbands you press when you find yourself alone on the floor in your home and you are unable to get up. You push the button and it generates an automatic call to a friend or neighbor, or 911.

Elders with limited incomes cannot afford these alert systems. So, here's my idea. If you need it, get a fall risk device for yourself and then agree to pay the monthly fee for someone else who cannot afford it. If you decide to do this, or something similar, I don't think you should call it "resilience." I think you should call it "wonderful." And by the way, Medicare does not cover this cost, but it should.

THREE

IDEAS THAT HEAL

Healing isn't about changing who you are. It's about changing how you feel about who you are.
—Suzanne Heyn

How We Age: Let's Start at the Bottom
Can You Hear Me Now?
Broken Hearts
The Flashing Yellow Light
Yawning Has a Story
Savor The Flavor
Gratitude Power
Wash Them
Six Word Stories
Rest Well, My Friend
Tidying Up
Make Way for the Robots

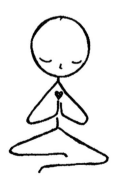

HOW WE AGE: LET'S START AT THE BOTTOM

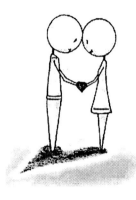

Exactly how do we age? The most referenced explanation (there are dozens) is called the "wear and tear theory." A reliable text on the physiology of aging defines it as "an accumulation of injuries and damages to parts of the body" resulting from periodically occurring, random impacts, i.e., use/overuse, accidents, disease, toxins, etc. This seems like a reasonable explanation. I get it.

Experts say, "Human beings fail the way all complex systems fail, randomly and gradually." We're designed with multiple layers of back-up (redundancy); we have an extra lung, an extra kidney, and extra teeth. But eventually one too many joints are damaged, one too many arteries calcify, and there are no more back-ups. We are worn down, or as one elder who is also a geriatrician (a medical doctor specializing in aging) puts it, "We just fall apart."

"Falling apart" happens in obvious and not-so-obvious ways. For example, we get gray hair, thinner hair, too. Our noses get wider and longer; our ears get bigger (honest, this is science-based). These are examples of age-related changes we cannot control.

But there are age-related changes we can control or, better put, "manage optimally." I'll start from the bottom. Feet get lots of wear and tear, after all. Are you giving your feet enough attention?

Little things like clipping your toenails regularly (is this too personal?) and having pedicures (both men and women can do this) are important, but always in salons with hygienic and well-kept soaking tubs. What about regular podiatrist or foot care visits. These are definitely worth considering.

Okay. Let's really get to the bottom of this. Take your shoes off and pull one of your feet up close for better viewing. Go ahead, just do it. Then take a close look at the other foot.

Your next steps will probably be fairly obvious. Take them, please.

CAN YOU HEAR ME NOW?

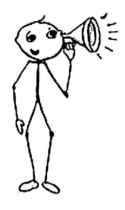

Here's the scene. I'm sitting in the driver's seat of my car in the shadiest spot possible at Costco's parking lot. I've not started the car's engine yet—I'm reflecting on what just happened to me.

Instead of an automobile packed with open-top cardboard boxes containing enough groceries and household items to last a month or more, I have one small white bag sitting on the seat next to me.

Something else is different, too. In and behind each ear, I have a hearing aid. It took me almost fourteen months from the date of my initial appointment for a hearing evaluation to get to this moment of actually acquiring hearing aids.

I usually make decisions quickly, but I kept putting this one off. *"After all,"* I told myself, *"a 'mild to moderate' hearing loss justifies waiting. Then there's the cost to be considered."* Hearing aids are an investment, and caring for them seemed like just another thing I would have to remember to do.

I've been awash in reasons for procrastinating. I had a difficult time envisioning tiny plastic and wire contraptions attached to my ears. I recalled the difficulties my mother had getting batteries into her hearing aids. But perhaps the biggest reluctance was the bold and highly public statement they make about getting old. Not that I think acknowledging age is a bad thing. But hearing aids are things grandparents wear—but wait, I *am* a grandparent.

As I sit in my car, using the rearview mirror to determine how visible these lightweight devices are in my ears and checking to assure that one did not already fall out, I feel exhilarated. Yes, that's the word. Mission accomplished—new horizons beckon.

After all, I was having trouble hearing questions when I taught classes or gave presentations. And when my soft-voiced granddaughters visited, I kept asking them to repeat their comments to the point I was fearful they would stop making them.

So here I am—minutes into a new way of engaging the world. I'm aware of the cacophony of noises around me. I'd become totally adjusted to my hearing loss and now I am realizing there are sounds I'd not heard for years. The crinkling of the paper bag containing all my hearing aid paraphernalia is incredibly loud (the hearing specialist said this would be the case and perhaps the most difficult sound to adjust to) but the birds chirping in a nearby tree are a delight. There's also the joyous sound of children laughing as they pass my parked car.

I start the engine and back out of the lot. As I make the turn and exit onto the highway, I am struck by a loud clicking sound. No wonder people riding with me always kept reminding me to turn off the blinker. My new hearing aids allow me to hear something I have never heard before—and our car is six years old!

Notice how possessive I have already become. I just referred to them as *my* hearing aids.

BROKEN HEARTS

 I had always suspected there was something called "broken heart syndrome," but I never anticipated finding research to support it. But, there it is. Reliable data indicating emotional stress can actually cause heart failure.

The nineteen aging individuals in the study I'm referring to have no previous indication of heart problems. However, they had all recently experienced a stressful event, after which they displayed chest pain, shortness of breath, and/or lightheadedness. Echocardiograms (tests using sound waves to view the pumping heart) confirmed the diagnosis. Each person was indeed having a heart attack.

The stressful events were not always situations you might expect. Of course, there were circumstances involving the death of a loved one, robberies, car accidents, or fierce arguments. But there were some joyful reunions and parties where it did not seem likely stress would occur, but it did.

According to researchers at Johns Hopkins University and Harvard Medical School, these nineteen people were studied over a four-year period. In each case, a significant stressful situation occurred, followed by a heart attack within twelve hours.

This research reminded me how important it is to understand and manage stress, especially as we age, because there's a lot more of it. As we get older, we experience significant losses (careers, spouses, reduced vision, and diminished hearing). We're also expected to deal with incredibly dramatic transitions. I'm thinking of my friend Delores, who went from her cozy little home into the hospital and then to a four-bed rehab unit. From there, it was back to the hospital and then to another rehab unit—all within a month's time. This is stressful.

I'm actually becoming a little agitated just recalling Delores and what happened to her.

Last week I had a conversation with a cool-headed, warm-hearted, seventy-nine-year-old fellow who seems to have all this figured out, and he's helping other folks do the same. He's a well-trained, volunteer peer counselor who works in personally innovative ways to provide supportive services to older adults. People like this exist in most communities. You might have to look around a little, but then again your next-door neighbor might intuitively have the right kind of skills and be very interested in talking and listening.

Aging individuals with emotional difficulties are a stoic lot. They often suffer silently. Folks in their seventh decade and beyond don't like to talk about their problems with just anyone. When they do discuss personal issues, they often prefer to talk with someone similar to them in age and experience. What an honor to be that person. It's not every day you get invited to heal a broken heart.

THE FLASHING YELLOW LIGHT

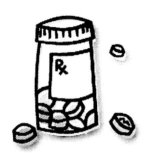

Consider the words that follow a flashing yellow light. As we age, medications become a significant part of our lives. Medical conditions that caused our grandparents' deaths are now easily treated with a simple prescription. We are blessed with availability and burdened with an overwhelming array of pills.

As we add years, we are more at risk of experiencing problems with medications. Older people are more likely than any other age group to have one or more chronic diseases. Multiple diseases can mean multiple medications and complex dosage schedules. Normal aging alters the way these medications are absorbed and metabolized in our bodies. Sometimes the effect is insignificant. Sometimes it can be dramatic.

Research suggests that at least fifty percent of people who take medications do not take them correctly. The examples include thinking "more is better" or dealing with a forgotten dose by doubling the next dose.

In the years before her death, my aunt took fourteen medications every day. Her life was shaped by the need to take a particular pill at a designated time. Her medications were organized in a multi-compartment, plastic container marked with the hours of the day. She identified each medication bottle with descriptive words like "pain" or "sleep" to protect against confusion. Wisely, Aunt Ethel was on a first name basis with her local pharmacist. She carried a pharmacy printout of all her medications in her purse, and took it with her when she saw her health care provider.

After some rather heavy-duty lobbying by me, Aunt Ethel knew she should take her pills with water and not a cup of coffee. There was notable potential for an adverse drug reaction with the number of pills she had been prescribed, and taking them with anything but water only added to the risk.

The risk of adverse reaction increases dramatically with each medication taken. Pharmacists tell me if you take eight or more medications (over-the-counter medications and herbal teas should be included in this count) your risk of interaction and resulting complications is nearly 100 percent.

I am advised that drug reactions often mimic signs or symptoms of other diseases, which means staying vigilant to any change in elder behavior. For example, mental confusion, which is sometimes misdiagnosed as a sign of Alzheimer's disease or another form of dementia, could be caused by medications taken for heart problems.

Today's medicines have tremendous benefits. They cure disease, help manage symptoms, reduce pain, and speed recovery. But along with the benefits, some medications carry risks, and all medications can produce undesirable side effects. Remember the reference to the flashing yellow light? The best protection is basic knowledge. Know what pills you are taking. Quiz both your doctor and your pharmacist. For example, say something like, "You said take two before bed? Is that just before I go to sleep or right after supper?"

I had selfish motives for my level of concern about medication management for my Aunt Ethel. I was planning a truly gala celebration for her ninetieth birthday. She made it to the party and lived well beyond that date. I am going to take just a little bit of credit for making it happen.

YAWNING HAS A STORY

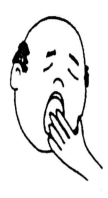 It's contagious. If you're sitting near someone who yawns, you will almost assuredly follow their lead. One study indicated fifty-five percent of people yawn within five minutes of seeing another person do it. Blind people yawn after hearing someone yawn. Babies yawn in the womb. Just typing the word "yawn" makes me feel inclined to open wide, drop my jaw a bit, and breathe in deeply through my nose.

Okay—I'm done. The typical yawn lasts about six seconds, but mine actually seemed longer. What is all this about anyway? Yawning is a message—at least that's what I've always believed. For example, if I'm presenting information to a group and several people in the audience start yawning, I get the message. Or do I?

The most-often-held science-based theory, which is not based on any science at all, is that a yawn replenishes our oxygen level. The idea that yawning is a way for the body to take in more oxygen is untested. Although, I do think it meets the test of common sense.

Tests are definitely underway about yawning, and they seem promising. There's a theory put forward by a father-son team at the University of Albany (Andrew and Gordon Gallup). They say, "Yawning cools the brain." Their belief is "Our brains are like computers, they only operate efficiently and effectively when they're cool."

According to these researchers, yawning reinstates optimal mental functioning. Now, if I carry this particular finding to its extreme, it means when I'm presenting information to a group and someone in the audience yawns, I should take it as a compliment. They're not bored—they're, in fact, so interested in what I'm saying they want to enhance the ability of their brains to process it.

There are many ways of thinking about this. There's another body of research that says sex is the reason we yawn, and that yawning has an erotic side. I briefly considered giving you more details about this area of study, but my "cooler head" prevailed. Yup, I'll let you pursue that one on your own.

There are many theories. Perhaps people yawn because they want to show off their straight, white teeth. Or how about this: baboons open their mouths wide and bare their teeth (yawn) in order to threaten their enemies. I've not found this applies to yawning behavior in humans, but if someone happens to look you in the eye and then opens wide and growls deeply, I suggest you don't stick around to inquire as to whether it's yawning behavior. Have you felt any urge to yawn in the last few minutes? (I'm just checking.)

Superstitions about yawning abound. It's suggested some people yawn when storms approach. There's also the theory that yawning is an indication of the "evil eye" (Greece), or that a yawn means someone is talking about you (Latin America, East Asia, and Central Africa). The ancient Greeks and the Mayan culture believed a yawn was an indication that someone's soul was trying to escape.

Here's my theory. I yawn when I'm tired. A nap usually follows. Speaking of escape . . . .

SAVOR THE FLAVOR

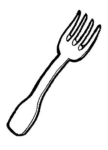 Are you ready? I have good news and bad. Research suggests Americans gain about a pound of weight during the winter holiday season. This is good news, because in the past we've heard that average weight gain is much higher (five to ten pounds) between Thanksgiving and Christmas Day.

But here's the bad news—really bad. Weight gained over the winter holidays isn't lost during the rest of the year. Let's say, we overeat at Thanksgiving and into the Christmas season and gain weight. But maybe we're more active in the spring and probably eating less mashed potatoes with gravy and fewer pieces of pie, so we lose some of the weight. This is good. But apparently about one pound a year of holiday eating, starting at about age forty, stays on our behinds and thighs until at age seventy . . . well, you get the picture.

Weight we pick up during the festive-eating season hangs around our hips and mid-section, gradually adding to our bulk—slowly but surely into the indefinite future. Year by year, it affects how we look and feel, and it has the potential to create significant mobility challenges and disease complications in later life. This reality came upon me like a small epiphany while I was preparing to facilitate a discussion on arthritis management. I became vividly aware of the direct relationship between the complications of arthritis and the extra weight we carry on our bodies.

Let me quote from a Johns Hopkins University publication that focuses entirely on arthritis. "There is an overwhelming association between Body Mass Index (the best indicator of overweight) and significant knee, hip, and back pain."

Here's the most important finding—the really good news. It does not take very much weight loss to decrease your risk of problems with arthritis. According to the Johns Hopkins publication, "Studies show that overweight or obese women who lose as little as eleven pounds cut their risk of knee osteoarthritis in half."

So . . . are you still with me? I'm not suggesting you avoid mashed potatoes and gravy forever and lose eleven pounds as soon as possible. I am suggesting that this year, for a change, you avoid gaining that extra pound. Weigh yourself right now and proceed as follows.

Have colorful healthy snacks readily available in a front-and-center area of your refrigerator over the next month. And remember, carrot, celery, and green pepper sticks can be as easily dipped in hummus as they can ranch dressing. If you're going to be a guest somewhere, make your dish-to-pass a healthy one. Once you arrive at the table, scan the food options before digging in. Prioritize. If you don't absolutely love something—don't eat it. Savor flavors. Take small portions—and the recommendation to chew each bite of food twenty to thirty times is definitely worth considering.

How about this idea? One healthy eating expert encourages us to, "Party hard during a holiday season, but focus on family, friends, and activities, rather than food." Savor the flavor of friendship.

GRATITUDE POWER

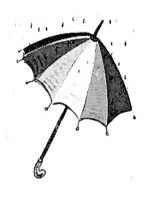

Do you believe in convergence? Think of it as a series of random encounters with a common theme. Maybe you recognize these events as a personal message, and maybe your behavior changes as a result.

Let me start at the beginning. A Florida State University study examined the power inherent in expressing gratitude. The experimental group (they were all romantic partners or best friends) was asked to make specific efforts to express appreciation—out loud. A control group was asked to freely recall pleasant memories, but told not to voice any appreciation. At the end of the three weeks, the people in the group that made acknowledging comments aloud rated their relationships as "stronger."

"True appreciation is an invitation." This phrase was printed in a Kansas State University Extension faculty newsletter encouraging more outright expressions of gratitude. It delineated the specific steps involved in using affirming comments, i.e., complimenting folks more often.

It begins with valuing what another person has done for you. For example, a woman I knew only through email exchanges picked me up at the airport after a long cross-country flight. Not only was she there when I got off the plane on a late Sunday evening, but she had an umbrella for me because the next day's forecast was rain and she knew I would be exposed to the elements. "Thank you!" was my response. But I could have done better. I could have said more.

For example, "Joan, I greatly appreciate your thoughtfulness. You met my plane, provided me with an umbrella I might need, and you were incredibly gracious. I'm so thankful to you." (It didn't rain, after all, and I'm thankful for that, too.) The reference materials on this topic suggest it's important to be both timely and authentic with expressions of gratitude. Use an engaging tone and smile when you offer up compliments.

I would like to add the idea of using an "I" message. Think about it. Let's say you encounter a friend who looks particularly fetching. You might say, "I like the periwinkle blue color of the dress you're wearing. It brings out the blue in your eyes." Or you could say, "You look nice." Both of these authentic acknowledgements are good, but the first one is so much better because you are speaking from the heart. Start with "I" and dress up (so to speak) your comments a little. When gratitude is expressed well and clearly, the person giving it experiences a sense of self-satisfaction, and the person receiving the compliment enjoys a huge boost to self-esteem.

My personal encounter with the role of well-expressed appreciation (i.e., the originally referenced study and the umbrella moment) can be called a "convergence." It made me want to offer more acknowledgements to people I care about (make that "people in general"). So I decided to spend a day acknowledging things I'd previously let pass without comment. I pledged to say "thank you" more frequently on that day and use individually-affirming "I" messages at every opportunity. And you know what? I had an absolutely wonderful day. Want to give it a try?

Oops, poor modeling. Let me restate. "I'd be so grateful if you'd spend just one day stating heartfelt appreciation to people you care about."

Gratitude becomes you.

WASH THEM

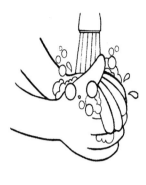

Permit me to tell you a story about hand-washing that might prompt you to do more of it.

Prior to the mid-1800s, hand-washing was not only ignored, it was soundly ridiculed. A Hungarian physician, Ignaz Semmelweis (later referred to as the "father of antiseptic procedures") protested loudly in favor of cleanliness, placing particular emphasis on the importance of hand-washing in hospital settings.

But the concept continued to be rejected by the public and physician colleagues. Ultimately Dr. Semmelweis was dismissed from hospital employment because of his unwavering position that hands must be washed well. He continued to advocate loudly for hand-washing (with a chlorinated lime solution) and public and professional reaction continued to be dismissive. In fact his ideas were so resoundingly rejected, he was declared insane and committed to a mental asylum. (Honest, I got this from a very reliable source.)

Today's physicians and surgeons would probably have their mental status questioned (or worse) if they did not adhere to hand-washing protocols. Here's a case in point. At Walter Reed Army Hospital in Washington D.C. every department in the hospital has a hand-washing monitor, i.e., someone who conducts passive surveillance and measures adherence to hand hygiene standards.

As older adults, we are in particular need of hand-washing rigor. As we age we are more vulnerable to infection. Our immune systems are more easily impacted by bacteria on something we have touched or by someone who has touched us. We have the potential to become ill more easily than we did as young and middle-aged adults, and we might not display the typical signs of infection (such as a high fever) until we become seriously ill.

Here's a simple but powerful infection control suggestion. If you find yourself or someone you love in a hospital setting, ask all of the hospital staff treating you, and any visitors to your hospital room, to wash their hands for 15 – 20 seconds with soap and warm water, and lots of friction. Request they do this before touching you (hugs included). I know, it seems excessive and you might be reluctant or even unable to make this request. But maybe you (or someone who cares about you) could place a little sign by your hospital bed asking that everyone do this—put a little happy face on the sign.

I think you can expect your health providers will wash often and well. But you might need to remind them. Smile when you make your request. For those loving, non-medical types who hover nearby when you're ill and provide comfort and support, don't hesitate. Prompting friends and family to get used to washing well might give them a better chance of staying infection-free when it's their turn to be hospitalized.

SIX WORD STORIES

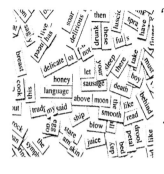

"Some believe it is only great power that can hold evil in check, but that is not what I have found. It is the small everyday deeds of ordinary people that keep the darkness at bay. Small acts of kindness and love."

This quote is from J.R.R. Tolkien, author, poet and philologist. In his book *The Hobbit*, these comments are offered as an explanation as to why the wizard (Gandalf) selected a small hobbit (Bilbo) to accompany the dwarves to fight the enemy. "Philology," by the way, can be loosely defined as "the study of language to determine its meaning."

In times past, I recall witnessing fervent discussion among fans of Tolkien's high-fantasy writings. In one instance, they explored the use and intention of these particular words; it was actually mesmerizing. But I choose to take the statement as it stands and simply let it be a reminder of the power and value of small and affirming actions.

I would never describe myself as a philologist, but I was once referred to as a "word merchant," and I relish well-stated phrases that carry positive imperative. The year ahead appears to be a time when public discourse is going to continue to be fiery and reactive. As a result, it will also be a time when small acts of kindness and love are more needed than ever before. At this writing, I am fantasizing that if we all put forth daily moments of truth and acknowledgement that are reflective and not reactive, we might fuel an epidemic of goodwill.

This brings me to the central idea in this essay. I offer you a tool that promotes and encourages small acts of kindness and love. Or maybe it's a way to corral and redirect reactive dialogue. My plan is to encourage your use of "the six-word story" to affirm and describe a life experience or vent a feeling you hold—in a constructive manner. Are you inclined to go dark and be negative? Please try not to do that. Try to use six words positively.

The original six-word story is attributed to Ernest Hemingway. His words "For Sale, Baby Shoes, Never Worn" might resonate with some readers. Whether Hemingway was the first person to use this method of telling a tale or some other writer can claim attribution, it's an approach much favored by teachers of writing over the decades. Maybe it's a distant cousin of Twitter? Some say it's an extraordinary oversimplification of Haiku.

But let it be your turn. See if you can come up with six words to describe the past year. Maybe it will be something like this: "Tough Year. Lost Hope. Found It."

I recently saw a seasonal posting. "The holidays are over. Thank God." And another one stood out. "I ordered a smile to go." And yet another six word story. "I often stumble, but rarely fall." Make your own six word stories. Try to go high, not low.

REST WELL, MY FRIEND

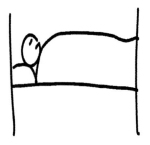

I have a few questions. Did you sleep well last night? Did you get seven to nine hours of restorative rest and wake up refreshed? Any interesting dreams? I've found when I pose such questions to people my age and older, there's frequently a head-shaking sigh. Sometimes I get a growly "Didn't sleep a wink" response.

So, let's look more closely at this business of a good night's sleep. Being well rested is essential to how we function on any given day. It's important that no matter what our age and how difficult to achieve, we need to be well rested, especially as we get older.

An optimal night's sleep enhances the functioning of our immune system, which helps stave off the increasing likelihood of age-related illness and disease. And this should get your attention—sleep actually improves memory, especially if we dream. It contributes to our ability to focus and concentrate.

Just as a drill, ask someone whose memory you admire (that friend of yours with an unfailing recall of names, perhaps) how she slept last night. Get personal. When I did this with a particularly well-rested elder, she told me she reads herself a bedtime story—out loud. She keeps some of her grandchildren's picture books near her bed and "practices" reading to herself in preparation for their next visit. Love that idea!

But maybe you need more than a bedtime story. If you want better rest, perhaps you should examine the reasons behind your inability to sleep. Are you eating too much rich, spicy food during the day or drinking alcohol too close to bedtime? Are you not getting enough exercise throughout the day? Regular, structured exercise is critical to sleeping well, but many experts suggest at least a six-hour window between any kind of vigorous physical activity and climbing into bed.

Sleeping poorly can be directly related to the side effects of some of the medications we take. Ironically, sleep can also be impacted by the pain we have when we don't take these same medications. Pain is, in fact, one of the biggest reasons for not sleeping well. Sometimes just switching the time of day you take a particular pill can make a huge difference in how well you rest that night. Query your physician or pharmacist before you make any changes.

I've looked at several sleep disorders studies, and the most common cause of sleeping difficulties is poor sleep hygiene; this includes absent or ineffective sleep rituals, or a less than ideal nighttime environment. There is an array of research-based recommendations on this topic. The ideas include getting sunlight a couple of hours each day to help regulate sleep-wake cycles. Some of these experts also suggest keeping a sleep diary and using it to track lifestyle changes and recent stressors.

But here's my favorite approach. University of Maryland researchers call it "quiet ears." Tonight, when you climb into bed, lie on your back, eyes closed, with your hands behind your head in a relaxed position. Place your thumbs in your ears closing your ear canal. Yes, really . . . try this. I know it seems silly, but it actually works. When you have both thumbs in your ears, you'll hear a high-pitched rushing sound (this is normal). Lay quietly listening to the sound for 15 – 20 minutes. Then put your arms down at your sides, take a deep breath, and go to sleep. Pleasant dreams.

TIDYING UP

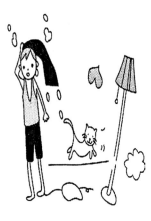

Stuff happens. I'm referring to all the miscellaneous vases, unmatched plastic containers, and outdated magazines—those various and assorted items you have accumulated over the years. Does your home have overflowing closets, overstuffed drawers? Is there any chance you can barely squeeze your car into the garage because of the precariously high piles of things on the floor? Did you say you can't get the car in your garage at all?

Is it wearying to think of what to do about all your stuff? Of course it is.

I have a solution that can help you manage your excess of material possessions forever. That's the promise made in the book *The Life-Changing Magic of Tidying Up: The Japanese Art of Decluttering and Organizing*, researched and written by the unexpectedly provocative clean-up expert Marie Kondo. It has some interesting new angles on this business of over-the-years accumulation of "stuff."

Let me begin with full disclosure. I am a relatively neat person. I was always a little impatient with my mother's tendency to hang on to so many things she didn't seem to need. Her apartment was full of ceramic figures of all shapes and sizes, and shelves of dusty books. I had a brilliant idea. "Mom, why don't you give one of your keepsakes away to someone every day. Choose who you want to receive the gift and I'll help you make it happen." She loved the concept, but she had so many possessions that we barely made a dent. When she died a year later, in my grief or because I didn't know what to do with her "keepsakes," I rented a storage unit and kept it for three years—visiting occasionally, always thinking my siblings might come and help me sort through her remaining things, I guess. They never did.

I'm reading Marie Kondo's book about tidying up on my Kindle so I don't add another book to our still-too-large collection of reading materials. Her basic premise is: "Keep things because you love them; keep only those items that give you real joy." The author recommends making dramatic changes "all in one go" or "ikki ni" in Japanese; she frowns on the idea of a little at a time.

The book's primary recommendation is: "Declutter by category, not place." For example, take all your clothing from every closet and drawer—including that box of off-season clothes in the garage, and pile everything together on the floor. Pick up each item individually; touch it, smell it. Ask yourself, *Does this give me joy?* If the answer is "no," discard it. Focus on what you want to keep, not what you want to give away. Ask yourself, *Am I happy wearing clothes that don't give me pleasure?* The author contends that putting your house in order is transformative and helps us discover ourselves in new ways and identify what is truly precious.

It's such a simple question, "Does it spark joy?" As we age and encounter life's increasingly challenging questions, this might be one of the more important ones. I think it has much broader application than an organized closet.

MAKE WAY FOR THE ROBOTS

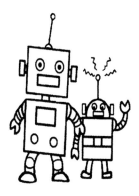

We call her "Alice." She's been with us for over two years—docked in our utility room and called upon to gather dog hair and dust from our floors on a daily basis. Her self-determined circling and bumping motions reassure me that the needed cleaning will get done and I do not have to do it. Alice travels room to room in our home as if on a mission. She is focused and intentional. I am occasionally amazed at what she vacuums up—and always appreciative when she does. An attempt at our dog's long, flopping tail—maybe not so much.

When Alice has exhausted herself in her efforts to keep our household intact, a pleasant female voice says, "Please charge Roomba," which is her original name. I immediately put her on the docking station, always marveling at the fact she said, "Please."

Alice aka Roomba was our first introduction to in-the-home "robots."

But then we met Alexa. She is billed as a "personal assistant" and advertised as Amazon Echo. Alexa is new on the market and quite popular during the holiday season, I am told. Alexa is a black, cylindrical, voice-activated "robot" that you link to your in-home Wi-Fi and then simply plug into an available outlet. She was a combined birthday and Christmas gift to my husband. He can be quite the skeptic and a hard man to shop for—and he really likes her.

It took about five minutes. Maybe it happened when he asked Alexa to play his favorite Glen Miller medley and she did so within seconds. It might have been when she knew the time of a televised football game he wanted to watch. Maybe it happened when I asked Alexa if she could "tell me the name of my husband" and she responded with, "I'm surprised you do not already have that information." We later found out that Alexa has a very well-defined sense of humor.

Seniors eagerly welcome battery-powered friends. Older adults stand ready to embrace technology. Not only do we welcome these new "friends," sometimes we become totally smitten. As the director of the AgeLab at the Massachusetts Institute of Technology puts it, "For too long technology has been chasing problems rather than trying to delight human beings." The next 5 – 7 years will be pivotal in terms of new technology being embraced by old people.

It's becoming clear that robots in some form can assist, educate, engage, and entertain older adults. Think about the possibilities. Robots could be used to help augment the adult caregiver role. They might positively impact isolation and loneliness. I envision robots that prompt people to take their medications in a timely fashion and encourage nutrient-dense eating. Robots you can snuggle exist in Japan. Therapy robots to help ease dementia symptoms are being studied. Robots that can lift and carry bed-bound elders when fatigued caregivers cannot are already a reality in some areas. I envision our neighborhood getting its own robotic helper someday soon. It will roll along our curb-cut sidewalks from house to house, engaging individuals and families. I'll check with the neighbors, of course, but I think "Mr. Rogers" would be an appropriate name.

FOUR

AGING IN PLACE: GET READY

I told the doctor I broke my leg in two places.
He told me to quit going to those places.
—Henny Youngman

Riddles
Staying Power
It's a Problem
Age-Friendly Audits
If You Are Going to Do It, Do It Right
Walk On By
CAPABLE
Has Health Gone Missing?
Hospitals
Invitation to an Obituary

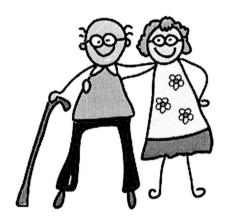

RIDDLES

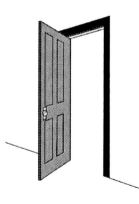

Here's a riddle for you. "What's black and white and red all over?" I'm sure you know the answer to this one. It's "a newspaper," of course. What about this one? "The more you take, the more you leave behind." Answer: "Footsteps."

Here's one that's a little trickier. "A man is trapped in a bathroom and the room has only two possible exits, two doors. Through the first door there's a room constructed from magnifying glass. The blazing hot sun immediately fries anything or anyone who enters. Through the second door there's a fire-breathing dragon. How does the man escape?"

I recognize this riddle is a bit over the top. But stay with me here; I'm trying to make a point you will remember forever. The answer to the last riddle is "The man waits until nighttime and then he goes through the first door." It's common sense, with a twist and a fire-breathing dragon. But perhaps the better question is this "How does someone get trapped in a bathroom?"

It can happen in a number of ways in real life. Let's say you're in a bathroom and you experience a stroke or heart attack—or maybe you just have a fainting spell. You're incapacitated and you drop down and slump against the door with a thud. When emergency help arrives, it becomes immediately apparent the door to that particular bathroom opens into the room itself and your somewhat bulky frame pressed against the door from the inside prevents a family member or a paramedic from easily entering to attend to you. You are trapped.

But you don't need to be. Check the direction your bathroom door opens and consider a simple turn-around to assure it opens out. Reverse the hinges and turn the door around. Voila! That's just one answer—I have loads of them.

The smallest room in the house can be a dangerous place. Bathrooms are hard-surfaced environments where water on the floor and soap in your eyes can lead to falls and fractures. The National Institute on Aging indicates "More than one in three seniors over age sixty-five falls each year, and eighty percent of falls occur in the bathroom." There are a multitude of unforgiving and slippery surfaces in a bathroom.

This is not a riddle. It's a reality that simple bathroom modifications hold the answer. Consider installing plenty of well-secured grab bars. Every bathroom needs vertical, horizontal, or angled bars positioned in a way that assures personal bathing and toileting experiences occur without mishap.

Most bathrooms could benefit from replacing the standard toilet with a comfort height toilet that's 17 – 19 inches high. A toilet riser is another approach. I have it on good report that Great Britain's King George II fell off the toilet and died as a result.

Dual head showers are available that glide down a vertical bar, making them easier to reach and maneuver when showering or bathing. Consider a shower chair, lights above the shower, levered door handles and faucets, and well-secured scatter rugs. My personal favorite is a one-handed toilet paper holder.

The bathroom is filled with ways to hurt yourself. Don't let this happen to you. This is not a joke.

STAYING POWER

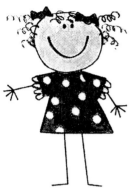

Did you know that 10,000 Americans turn sixty-five every day, and this will keep happening for well over the next decade? We are a force. The "oldest-old," people, eighty-five years and beyond, are the fastest growing segment in the population. Oh. My. Gosh.

Such staying power we have. This is also the name of a book by a Canadian author, Rachel Adelson. She advocates, "taking a new look at an old story" and chastises older adults (you, me, and our age peers) who succumb to what she calls the "ick factor." I had not heard this term used to refer to how one feels about aging. Actually, I found it off-putting.

But then, I realized even when I say, "I fully embrace aging," I don't always. There are some things about aging I don't like at all.

Achy knees are no fun. Trying to have a dinner conversation in a noisy restaurant with a husband who is unwilling to wear his hearing aids is definitely not pleasant. My inability to read the small print on a label to determine if the product contains the sodium that I'm not supposed to have too much of—again, no fun.

How do these predicaments make you feel about aging? Maybe getting your arms around this starts at home—after all, these are the environments in which we have a long history of control. They are also the places we might first notice that we have lost our independence.

"Aging-in-place" is the term used of late to denote staying power in your own home. We can practice dealing with our changing abilities in the privacy of our own bedrooms, bathrooms, and kitchens. I think we should grab control and really become a force in the world.

I have a host of ideas. Start by walking around your home and looking critically at what you see. Decide to "age-proof" your home. Try adding nightlights in bathrooms and hallways. Can you make them the kind that goes on automatically when the power goes out? Lever-style handles on doors would be useful, and maybe levered faucets, too. A handheld adjustable showerhead can come in quite handy.

Here's a personal example that speaks loudly. Opening cans and jars has become very difficult for me, of late. Arthritis in my thumbs and one wrist is the reason . . . I think. My frustration level mounts every time I try. I know this might sound a little strange, but purchasing an easy-use can opener in fire engine red has been my salvation. This colorful, ergonomically correct apparatus makes me feel better.

Sometimes I just lay it out on the counter in case I might need it while I'm cooking. Having it nearby makes me feel more in control, more independent. I do not even use it that much. I just like knowing I can. You are probably rolling your eyes at that last statement—but it's true.

My visiting daughter smiled and laughed at me when I told her my can opener story, and then she hugged me.

IT'S A PROBLEM

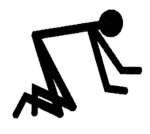

Every time an older adult walks on an uneven side-walk or steps onto a higher-than-usual curb, there can be a problem. It can happen when an aging person moves across an unsecured scatter rug wearing plastic-soled shoes. It's all about falling, or thinking you might.

A friend of mine (let's call her "Clara") fell and broke her hip. Not good at her age. But she's a strong woman, and I have faith she will prevail. What happened to her occurs more frequently than is commonly realized. The likelihood of falling increases dramatically with advancing age.

Another aging person I know (let's call her "Elise") also fell. She's a fragile ninety-two-year-old. She didn't break her hip, but something else happened. She developed a fear of falling, a very intense fear of falling.

Falls have a significant social and psychological consequence. People fall, or almost fall, and whether or not they sustain injuries, they develop a fear of losing stability. The National Council on Aging, Center for Healthy Aging, has comprehensively examined the available research on falling. They found fear of falling leads to lessened mobility, deteriorating health, a decline in physical and social functioning and, ultimately, nursing home admissions. Remember this is fear of falling; it's not even the actual fall.

Fear not. There are fall prevention strategies, and they are especially important if you know Clara or Elise or someone like them. Fall prevention starts with educating elders about risk. Those at high risk are typically over age eighty-five and have had two falls in the past year, or one fall with an injury, and/or a history of gait or balance problems.

If falling and possibly suffering a fracture are not something you want to experience, the single most effective intervention is exercise. It reportedly reduces the number of falls by almost twenty percent. Maybe your exercise of choice is Tai Chi. Perhaps it's balance, gait, or strength training. An exercise program doesn't mean you won't ever fall. It means reducing your risk and building your mobility confidence. It also means that if you do fall and a fracture results, you might have an easier recovery.

Do this, too. Get your vision checked so you can see those slippery scatter rugs. You probably know that any bathroom rug needs to have slip-resistant backing to protect you from falls, but have you looked at the wear and tear on that gripper-backing lately? Maybe the grip no longer grips? Maybe it never did. Just wondering.

Examine your medications, carefully considering the ones that make you feel unsteady, disoriented, or sleepy-headed. Talk to your doctor and/or your pharmacist about this.

Do what makes sense. This usually means taking an individually tailored approach that considers age, risk of falling, and personal/environmental factors. Are you now feeling a bit more educated about fall prevention? Please do one more thing, if you would. Educate someone else.

When you learn, you must teach.

AGE-FRIENDLY AUDITS

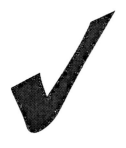

Some words are friendlier than others. For example, "genuine" is a beckoning word, don't you think? "Beneficial" is as well. One of the less friendly words in our language is "audit." For some, it calls up the vision of an IRS representative knocking loudly at the front door of your home.

I'd like to pose a different type of audit. It will always involve your front door, but it's genuinely beneficial. Age-friendly, if you will. I'm referring to a home audit to thoroughly assess your living environment in order to identify health and safety issues. Ideally, a trained observer who can offer possible solutions to any identified problems does it. But you could also do your own self-audit. The issues that surface during these in-the-home risk assessments, if not addressed and resolved, make it less likely you'll be able to age-in-place—which means living happily ever after in a home of your own.

Here's a preview of possible questions. Is your house number clearly visible from the street so an emergency vehicle can find you if they need to? Are your smoke and CO (carbon monoxide) detectors in working order? Do you even have a CO detector?

An in-home risk assessment can be thought of as "health insurance"—make that "assurance." Let me give you an example of potential impact. Many of the questions in an audit such as this focus on preventing in-the-home falls. New research indicates even if a fall doesn't land you in the hospital with an accompanying fracture, you might end up in the hospital for other reasons, including heart surgery or a colon resection. Having had a fall after a surgery is linked to post-operative complications.

In a large sample of older adults (average age seventy-four) who had one or more falls in the six months prior to surgery, a far greater percentage were found to have more post-operative complications (59 percent versus 25 percent in the colorectal group and 39 percent versus 15 percent in the heart surgery group). The folks with a fall history were more likely to be discharged to a rehab facility rather than to their homes after leaving the hospital and had a higher rate of hospital re-admission, as reported in an issue of the well-regarded American Medical Association journal, *JAMA Surgery*. For many health professionals, I hope this piece of information is an eye-opener that will launch further examination of ways to delay aging through preoperative risk assessments.

There are various home audit and risk assessment tools available. You might need to research it a bit. All of them promote an increase in healthy life years. Sounds beckoning, don't you think?

One more point. Credible analysis suggests an increase in healthy life years is estimated to have an economic benefit of $7.1 trillion dollars over the next five years. That's trillion with a "t."

I do not make this stuff up.

IF YOU ARE GOING TO DO IT: DO IT RIGHT

"Don't Fall for Me." As an educator, this is the name of a presentation I have given in senior centers, churches, and libraries over the last several years. I talk about fall risk and in-home fall prevention in practical and (as some kind person once told me) "very powerful" terms. If I could place a value on the impact of my words, I would estimate that each time I speak and there are ten or more people in the room, I save at least $30,000 in the societal and medical cost of falls and fractures. Hubris I know, but bear with me here.

I envision costs avoided and money saved, because each hospitalized fall costs more than $30,000 (Centers for Disease Control data, 2015) and I'm fairly positive that at least one person in my audience will harken to what is said and put simple in-home safety measures in play as a result. So much attention is given to being socially safe right now, so why not start at home.

That said I have a new angle on this topic. If you must fall—do it "the right way," Keep in mind that no matter what anyone says, one in three older adults will fall—with one in five of that number breaking something they would prefer were not broken—or experiencing a life-complicating head injury.

There's a "right way to fall." So say all the experts. My husband, who parachuted out of airplanes during his military training, and my brother, who was a helicopter firefighter for years, heartily agree. According to Dr. Jessica Schwartz, a physical therapist and fall expert, "It's almost inevitable you are going to fall, so you really should know how to do it."

Number one: Protect your head. If you don't, according to Dr, Schwartz, "You'll hit . . . like a coconut and get a concussion." This is definitely not a good thing. Many years ago, I fell off my bike while riding a little too fast over a gravely railroad trestle. The deep dent in my bicycle helmet that resulted said it all. Fortunately I was wearing a helmet.

The experts suggest that if you find yourself falling, do your best to pivot to your side and tuck in your head. Bend your elbows and knees, and try to take the hit in the fleshiest part of your body. A stuntman and assistant professor of acting, movement, and stage combat at the University of Wyoming, Kevin Inouye, says, "Aim for the meat, not the bone."

A decade ago, I fell when a heavy, fast-rolling cart knocked into my ankles and toppled me. I reached out with my hands to try to catch myself and broke my wrist. A wrist is "not forgiving" when you go down on it. The technician who put on my cast said, "You will probably have arthritis in that wrist as you age." And I do.

I am told the key is "don't fight the fall." Roll with it, like paratroopers do. As martial art instructors do. The best advice is don't fall, but if you do, do it right.

WALK ON BY

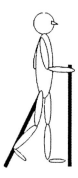I have a neighbor in her nineties who credits me with saving her life. She bases this observation on something I wrote several years ago about the critical importance of taking a brisk, aerobic walk for thirty minutes each day. She embraced the advice completely, and her blood pressure responded as if it had been ordered to do so.

I always thought my friend's reference to "lifesaving" was a little excessive, until I came upon a website that boldly stated she was right. An Internet-based article in "Next Avenue" encourages "grown-ups to keep on growing" and indicates walking twenty minutes every day can save your life. This doesn't mean you can't walk for thirty minutes; it just means you don't have to. www.nextavenue.org

Similar information came from another ninety-year-old walker named Barbara Knickerbocker Beskind, who was a participant in the 2015 Influencers in Aging Project. Barbara's advice is simple, "Stay vertical and moving forward . . . keep your ears over your hips and your hips over your heels." Can you see this? More importantly, will you do it?

Walking has enormous benefit. Current research suggests it affects our aging bodies emotionally and even creatively, in addition to the well-known benefits to the pulmonary and cardiovascular system. More often, it's suggested we walk using a pair of ski poles. They give us better stability. If your vision is declining, ski poles can help you remain aware of the terrain you're walking on and lessen the likelihood of any stumbling. After all, "face-to-sidewalk" moments are something we all want to avoid.

Ski poles might be exactly the thing that gets you out the door and moving. The vertical grip promotes good posture, in addition to the fact that using ski poles declares to anyone who happens to be watching that you're a healthy, and active ager—someone who is fully engaged in life. If the poles don't appeal to you, perhaps you can get better shoes.

Maybe you will become so enamored with the potentially powerful influence of a daily walk that you decide to acquire a pair of really good walking shoes before you head out the front door. Maybe you don those shoes and just walk around the interior of your home for twenty minutes? Either way, bulky and stiff sneakers are out—comfort is in. Be sure you get elastic laces because they are a cinch to tie. They stay tied but also allow you to slip off your shoes with ease when your health trek is over.

Scholarly articles regularly report that health-compromising behaviors such as physical inactivity are difficult to change. Let's say you read something touting the importance of a 20 to 30-minute walk. You're persuaded, and you say to yourself, *I can do that.* Then you don't.

But you're reminded of your promise when you see your aging neighbor stride by in her well-fitting walking shoes with ski poles firmly in hand. Her poles have little rocker bottoms (you can find them at sporting goods stores) and she actually seems to be floating.

She's modeling "best practice" aging, and her behavior has the likelihood of changing yours. Let it.

CAPABLE

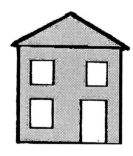

If someone told you that the home you live in (and want to remain in until the end of your days) could be made measurably safer, literally almost assuring your aging-in-place preferences can be realized, and at a relatively small cost, you would probably want to know more. Of course you would.

Here's the deal, or perhaps we can call it the beginning of an idea. A study completed at Johns Hopkins University School of Nursing referred to as CAPABLE (Community Aging in Place—Advancing Better Living for Elders) focused on innovative approaches to supporting older adults in living more comfortably and safely in their own homes. It started with a group of aging home dwellers who were given an in-home assessment of fall-risk potential and an evaluation of personal independence in activities of daily living (bathing, toileting, and dressing etc.).

In this study, an occupational therapist did a comprehensive in-the-home evaluation of problem areas and offered what were often seen as very simple recommendations. Then a licensed, bonded handyman (yes, it is a "handyman" we are talking about here!) made the recommended home modifications, including the installation of handrails or grab bars, the secured placement of a toilet riser, or the addition of an emergency light in the bathroom (or the hall going toward the bathroom). Each situation is different.

The CAPABLE results demonstrated an improved ability for independence and a greater capacity to age-in-place. Simple changes that are often very inexpensive can have measurable impact. Home safety assessment and modification appear to be "a very cost-effective health sector intervention." Targeting this type of intervention to older people with previous fall injuries is even more cost-effective.

To make my point further, here is another example. A randomized trial published in the *Journal of the American Geriatrics Society* found "interventions such as home modifications increased home safety." The cost for equipment and home modification, including devices, delivery, and installation is actually very low. Participants reported "significant improvements in the specific activities of daily living compared to the control participants, with the greatest improvements in bathing and toileting, as well as a decrease in home fall hazards."

When you are in a clinic talking with your health care providers, they have no idea there are piles of tipping-over newspapers and glossy (slippery) magazines on the floor beside your recliner. They don't know you have a suction cup grab bar in your bathing area, your porch light has burned out, and there's no battery in your smoke alarm.

Enter the handyman. Health professionals and insurers take note; harken to the possibilities.

HAS HEALTH GONE MISSING?

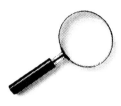 It feels like jumping into a fire pit, but I'm compelled by forces I cannot completely identify, to offer this: The word "health" seems to be missing in the discussions about any remodeling of our national health care system.

The dictionary defines "health" in one of two ways: (1) the state of being free from illness or injury, i.e., strength, vigor, wellness, and well-being or "fine fettle;" (2) physical or mental condition, i.e., "His mental health seemed precarious." Sometimes there's a third meaning and the word "health" is used to express friendly feelings toward one's companions while drinking.

If I continue to present this topic as forthrightly as I am envisioning, I might need that drink later—but let's continue. Once you have defined health, there are certain assumptions you must make about it. Assumption #1: It is in the best interests of our country that we have a healthy population, no matter what the age or circumstance. Healthy people are more productive.

Assumption #2: In today's world, people, healthy or not, live longer. In 1900, the average life expectancy was 47.3 years. In 2015, it was 71.5 years.

Which brings us to assumption #3: Longevity does not assume absence of disease. We are destined to live longer, but we will almost assuredly end up with a chronic disease such as a heart condition, diabetes, arthritis, or osteoporosis. As I have observed before, "Chronic diseases are like wolves, they travel in packs." Think about it like this, according to the National Council on Aging, ninety-two percent of adult over age sixty have one chronic condition; seventy-seven percent have at least two or more.

The fourth assumption is couched in my own perspective, but I think it's defensible. Achieving and maintaining good health, or managing a chronic condition once you have it, is pivotal in all this. It can be assumed that if people do not have access to health care or cannot afford health care, they will ultimately end up getting sicker and be more likely to land in expensive, high-dependency living situations.

High blood pressure, left untreated, can evolve into heart-related issues or stroke, which can require multiple medications, frequent hospitalizations, or invasive surgery. High blood sugars, unchecked, can lead to diabetic fragility with a greater likelihood of debilitating neuropathy and lost mobility. Let me be very specific and highly practical about the costs involved when we don't put "health" at the heart of our discussions. If we remodel our health care system without embracing that we have increasingly larger numbers of older, longer-living, potentially sicker people, we do so at societal peril.

We are smarter than that, aren't we? Aren't we?

HOSPITALS

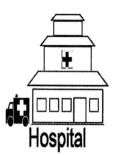

Hospital

As we grow older, the possibility of hospitalization increases. Falls are one of the biggest reasons. Despite loads of available advice about what we must do to avoid falling, it still happens. And when it does, you end up on the floor dazed and sometimes in excruciating pain. In all likelihood, 911 is called and paramedics appear; you travel by ambulance to an emergency room for assessment and x-rays—and you are (quite probably) placed in a hospital bed. So this is about hospitals.

In the recent past I've spent many hours in a hospital setting providing support to a beloved elder friend (his picture is on the cover of this book) who experienced a spectacular fall. He broke his femur, the biggest bone in the leg. He was playing a gig in a local senior center—saxophone in hand and a smile on his face—but he turned too quickly and lost his balance. I'd given him all my best information on fall prevention and he'd listened. But it still happened.

This man is an incredibly strong and smart elder who has a great attitude and a loving partner. After an impressive procedure involving pins and clips and skilled surgeons, he was able to bear his full weight in six weeks. Good news; good hospital.

Being admitted to a hospital has been referred to in the literature as similar to traveling in a foreign country. The sounds and smells are unfamiliar and the people you meet seem to speak another language. But that's where the comparison ends. Whether it's a planned trip or an emergency medical situation, the thought of hospitalization likely prompts trepidation and a sense of losing control, especially for older adults who might already be experiencing losses such hearing, vision, and a reliable sense of balance.

In a hospital situation, the first thing you lose is your clothes; in the case of falls and fractures, clothing sometimes has to be literally cut off your body. The hospital gowns you're given resemble being loosely wrapped in tissue paper, and not enough of it. You lose privacy, especially in a double room with only a thin curtain separating you and your roommate. You lose sleep because you're constantly being awakened for some procedure or another, after which you're told to "get some rest."

I could go on; there are other losses to catalog. But they're usually temporary. Let's focus on the gains. There is an interesting website sponsored by the National Transition of Care Coalition (www.ntocc.org), which provides guidelines on how to optimize a hospital stay. It reminds patients and their families to communicate symptoms as well as their feelings. It stresses the importance of having a list of current medications (prescription and non-prescription), which includes everything from what the pill looks like to the time of day you take it. A list of your medications is something you can control.

But here's the real take-away. Being in a hospital setting allows us to witness health care in action. It's incredibly impressive to see knowledgeable and well-trained medical professionals thoughtfully teaming with one another in a patient-focused fashion. New treatment options go beyond what I thought was possible—way beyond, and care is provided in a sensitive and personalized manner.

No wonder there's such uproar in this country over health care. It's personal. It's life-saving. It's definitely not something we want to lose.

INVITATION TO AN OBITUARY

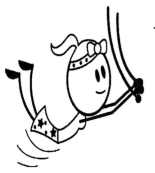

It's a typical Sunday evening in the Johnson household. There's a thin crust, spinach-garlic pizza in the oven delivering its incredible aroma throughout the house. My husband and I are having a glass of wine and playing a game of scrabble on my iPad. He's winning.

I've been pondering the idea of posing something a little out of the ordinary to him and decide this might be the moment to broach it. So I say, "How about a little later tonight, or maybe tomorrow night, you and I write our obituaries?" He stops, mid-Scrabble play, and looks at me incredulously as if to say, *Who are you exactly?*

Well . . . I'm a seventy-something woman who reads the obituaries regularly. I'm especially fond of the ones with a photograph where the person looks close to their age at the time of death, and I like casual photos in which the person is smiling widely. Don't we all want to be remembered smiling? I prefer obituaries that identify the cause of death. This is pure curiosity on my part, I suppose. I also like a little lightheartedness—the deceased person's favorite color possibly? I can imagine an obit that includes something like, "His favorite color was plaid and he loved a tall glass of tomato juice with buttermilk in the late afternoon, mixed together, equal portions of each." Words like these should have been in my father's obituary, but there were none. And I'm a little sad about it.

But, I digress—let me return to my original query. I tell my still-wide-eyed husband I read an obituary recently that was written by the deceased person before her death. I found it "charming," which is not a word typically used to describe the narrative outlining someone's life and recent death. But it fits. The woman's name was "Sharon," same name as mine, which might explain my resonance with what she did and my interest in replicating it. She used simple, tender words to describe her happy life, and she encouraged the reader to honor her death by performing "an act of unexpected kindness." Lovely request—don't you think? I did exactly what she asked that very day, and the next day as well.

I'm not the first person to think about writing an obituary in advance of death. I tell my still-listening husband there's even a template to help us get us started: www.obituaryguide.com. I remind him we feel good about the other things we have done related to end-of-life planning that opened our eyes to the critical importance of open-hearted and thoughtful conversations about death and dying.

I'm going on and on and my husband is warming to the obituary preparation idea, I think. He suggests we continue this discussion later. Okay. I'm in no rush. It's the kind of writing one gives a lot of thought. I want it to be unforgettable.

FIVE

WHAT IF YOU DON'T REMEMBER WHAT YOU FORGOT?

*One of the best things about aging is being able to
watch imagination overtake memory.*
—Harriet Doerr

Waiting to Be Remembered
I Remember When . . . But Do I?
The Thing We Forget With
Living in the Age of Distraction
Memory Palace
Check. List.
Plastic Brains?
Our Greatest Fear

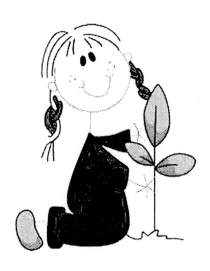

WAITING TO BE REMEMBERED

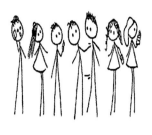

Forget something? Me too. I've had a lot on my mind lately, and when this happens, I get really forgetful. Last week I arranged to be in two places at once. I left my purse in a restaurant. And, this is fairly embarrassing; I was asked a simple grandmotherly kind of question and I could not remember my youngest granddaughter's middle name. I had to look it up. (Fortunately, I did recall where to look.)

No, I don't have early-stage dementia. It's just simple forgetting. It happens to all of us, and it happens more often as we age. When I'm extremely busy with life, it happens a lot. My favorite comment from a gerontologist friend of mine is, "Your brain is like a library. An old library has more books—so it takes longer to retrieve one." This little phrase gives me a tremendous amount of personal comfort.

Memory difficulties accompany aging. According to researchers at Johns Hopkins University, at least fifty percent of people over fifty have some degree of simple forgetting, Even so, the out-of-control, forgetting-something-important experience can be extremely unsettling.

I believe I know what causes my memory lapses. I call it "stimulus overload," too much on my mind, a lifestyle issue. I'm sometimes surprised people don't realize how the things we do, or don't do, can make a big difference in how often we misplace an object or forget the name of someone close to us. For me, overload is a major component.

Other lifestyle issues could be in play. Memory problems can be related to sleep (not enough of it) or physical activity (not enough of it) or food (not enough of the right kind). A new medication might explain why your Aunt Agnes is disoriented, when she used to be "as sharp as a tack." Familial expectations can play a role. For example, "Oh those Johnsons, they're always a little forgetful in their old age."

The reasons behind age-related memory problems can come in many forms. There is seldom just one explanation. Here's another consideration: memory problems can be undiagnosed depression. It caught my eye years ago, when a Stanford University Professor said, "When a patient comes in and complains about their memory, they're depressed until proven otherwise."

But it's the "what you eat, or don't" issue that gets most of my attention lately. In a highly credible, multi-year study, Dutch scientists found that folic acid (foliate), a B vitamin present in some grains and in dark-colored vegetables, can help memory. "Help" is an understatement. The research study showed this little powerhouse of a vitamin, available in vitamin pill form and in a variety of foods, has a dramatic and positive affect on cognitive ability.

Food sources include dark green leafy vegetables, beans and legumes, fruits (particularly citrus), wheat bran and chicken liver. These foods are sitting right there on our grocery store shelves, just waiting to be remembered.

I REMEMBER WHEN . . . BUT DO I?

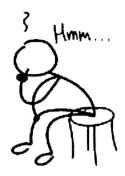

Does this happen to you? You start a task and get distracted and what you intended to do totally escapes your consciousness. Yesterday I stood in the hallway for a full minute with a bottle of spray cleaner in my hand trying to remember what I intended to clean. Then I realized I had just cleaned a surface in the kitchen and was in the process of putting the bottle away.

Maybe it happens this way. I'm trying to remember something, the title of a movie or the name of an old friend, and I just cannot do it. It's frustrating and unsettling. I struggle, take a few deep breaths, and it might eventually come to me—or it might not.

A long-ago article on the American Psychological Association's (APA) website was comforting. The statement said, "For the human brain, there's no such thing as over the hill." We all tend to forget more things as we age; it's disconcerting, but it's to be expected. Excessive worrying does not help.

Apparently, in the aging brain, *episodic* memory such as: "What did I have for breakfast?" and *source* memory: "Where did I learn about that new car" decline the most notably. *Semantic* memory, i.e., words, facts, and concepts, are less likely to be problematic. *Procedural* memory, for example: "knowing how to ride a bicycle" shows even less decline. *Implicit* learning, which is learning without conscious effort, seems to be mostly spared into old age.

Truth be told, I had a birthday recently and I forgot how old I was. A friend asked me and I gave myself a year beyond my actual age. I woke up in the middle of the following night realizing what I'd said, and I felt a little foolish (and slightly amused). I think I smiled and went back to sleep, which was a good thing, because getting enough rest is critical to older adult memory.

So is nutrient-dense eating (fruits, vegetables, and seafood). In recent weeks, it's been hectic in our household and I have not been especially observant about how much sleep or exercise I get. I've definitely been making more cookies than salads.

This brings me to my reason for writing about this topic in the first place. I almost forgot. Memory aids are one of the important comforts for the aging brain. We probably all have our own methods. I have a structured "to-do" list that I attach to a clipboard—it makes me feel more in control to have my clipboard at-the-ready. The calendar on my iPad is a godsend, and the fact that I have an iPad at all and it's mounted on an easy-to-see stand on the kitchen counter (that would be the sparkly, just-cleaned kitchen counter) helps me remember what I forget. Usually.

THE THING WE FORGET WITH . . .

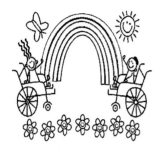

"Memory is the thing I forget with . . ." This is a child's definition of memory. The standard dictionary definition is "the power or process of reproducing or recalling what has been learned or retained." My favorite way of thinking about memory comes from Johns Hopkins University: "Memory is all the things you can remember and your capacity for remembering."

Our memory starts to change as early as age thirty. Here's an example from *Mental Fitness for Life* by Sandra Cusack and Wendy Thompson:

> *Now what's the name of that woman with the curly hair who's Susan's friend? I think her name begins with R or is it B? Rooster? No that couldn't be it—Brewster? Yes, that's it. And her first name? Is it biblical—Sarah? Rebecca? Judith? No, none of those. Elizabeth? Martha? Mary? I'm getting close. It's Mary something, Mary Anne? Mary Elizabeth? Oh wait; she has the same name as my granddaughter—Rosemary. No, not quite. But it does have a flower in it. Ah, it's Mary Rose. Mary Rose Brewster. At last!*

This problem occurs oh-so frequently for aging adults. It's referred to as the "tip of the tongue" syndrome. Has it ever happened to you? It happened to me just yesterday—twice.

If I forget the name of Susan's curly-haired friend and I really want to remember, it's more likely I'll remember if I focus on "pathways of association." The name of Susan's friend is stored somewhere in my memory, but it might not be where I thought it was. The process of trying to make the association means I'll use key words, sights, smells, sounds, and tastes, and any other available clues. It's both exhilarating and frustrating.

But here's the deal. The process of trying to recall something you've forgotten improves your memory. Yes, really. Even if I never make the association and ultimately have to ask Susan her friend's name, I'm better off cognitively because I struggled a little in trying to make associations.

Remembering things as we age gets increasingly more difficult. Understanding what gives us the most trouble can be useful. A Stanford University study (Von Lierer, et al) ranked the memory skills that people most want to improve:

1. People's names
2. Key dates and appointments
3. Location of household items
4. Recent and past events
5. When to take vitamins and medications, and
6. Important information and facts.

Consider this. Look at the areas listed in the preceding paragraph one more time. Rate your degree of difficulty in each category. Use a 1 – 5 scale that ranges from "seldom" to "always." For example, rating yourself as a "5" on "taking vitamins and medications" means that particular part of your daily activity is always challenging, and you'll need to be really creative about finding memory aids.

I would rate myself about a "3" in "ability to recall names"—sometimes I'm great at it; other times I draw a total blank. I have a friend who's a "5" in this category. For her, it's always been a significant problem.

But ultimately she solved it—and quite creatively. She just decided to start calling everybody "Sweetie."

LIVING IN THE AGE OF DISTRACTION

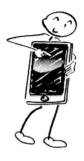

I will begin with full disclosure. I was in a conversation with someone recently about a topic with which I am totally familiar, and I was about to mention a fact I know quite well. A loud noise nearby caught my attention. Suddenly I could not remember the fact. *Breathe deep,* I told myself. *It will come.*

But it did not come. Well, ultimately it did. The next day I was talking with another person altogether on a totally different subject and I interrupted my own sentence to blurt out the earlier forgotten fact. It totally surprised the person I was talking with, and me, too.

Does this happen to you? Do you experience frustration when you attempt to recall something you know well but cannot remember? Distractions can make you go totally off-topic. Of course it happens to you. It happens to all of us.

Distractions that redirect a task or entirely hijack a situation can be particularly irksome. In an effort to better understand all this, I decided to Google "aging memory and distraction." I ignored the articles on miraculous memory-enhancing vitamins and focused on scholarly studies. I learned, or perhaps relearned, that distraction is a challenge to memory across the lifespan. It disrupts the ability to maintain a coherent stream of goal-directed thought and action at any age. This is comforting—I think. But these same academic sources state that as we get older, we definitely have more difficulty encoding and retaining relevant information. Our aging brains lose their filtering capacity.

I recall (and yes, I really do remember doing this) talking with my granddaughter about becoming distracted and forgetful sometimes. Her response was, "Oh Grandma, that happens to me all the time!"

We laughed together—it was an exchange I will never forget. Her tender acceptance of forgetful behaviors and a little laughter is not necessarily an evidence-based way of dealing with memory loss, but it sure works for me.

Researchers at the University of Southern California address aging cognition in plain speak: "The thing we are holding in our mind can be easily dislodged when our attention turns elsewhere." The intrusion of technology now makes this reality an even bigger problem for aging adults. Okay, I get it. The multi-tasking we are more and more prone to, such as listening to a riveting public radio program while cooking dinner, should be labeled a full-fledged interruption, not just a distraction, because of it's bigger impact overall.

My. Oh. My. This totally explains the unexpected presence of mandarin oranges in the shrimp and rice dish we had for dinner last night. It turned out to be quite delicious by the way. Maybe next time I'll add another kind of fruit and perhaps a little less cheese. But I digress.

I'm strangely comforted to find out I'm in league with my age peers in having issues with distraction. I'm also appreciative of knowing that my more frequent forgetting behaviors might be aided by a hard look at the possibly excessive presence of technology in my life. Now if I could just find my phone, everything would be fine.

MEMORY PALACE

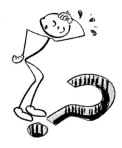

Have you heard of the "Memory Palace?" It's not a vacation spot on the coast or a just-in-time-for-the-holidays board game. It's a concept. It involves transforming what you want or need to remember into vivid mental images and then placing those images in a familiar architectural space.

Other than the business of getting old in the first place, which we all will (are), I continue to think memory loss (or worry about that possibility) is what concerns us the most as we move through the decades.

Enter an interesting approach to forgetting and remembering. It's sometimes called the "loci method," or even the "roman room technique," but I prefer "Memory Palace." This memory aid has been around for a really long time, but several memory experts are now discussing it more vigorously.

Let's say you have a busy day, with a variety of things to do. You need to call your sister, bathe the dog, pick up the dry cleaning, shop for a pair of boots, and bake a pumpkin loaf.

Let's begin, start like this. Envision your home. Imagine coming in the front door and standing in the foyer. Call that room #1. Now mentally walk through your home, numbering each room. Done? Okay. Next, using your mind, place a vision of each activity you want to do in a different numbered room. In the foyer, room #1, you might envision a huge telephone with a picture of your sister on all the dialing buttons (call your sister). In room #2 you might mentally place a white bath towel covered with dog hair in the middle of the floor (bathe the dog). In room #3 . . . well, I think you get the picture. It's all about creating pictures and mental images, and the more bizarre they are the better. Place the mental images, one-by-one, in a familiar environment and voila . . . easy recall.

I used this approach two weeks ago when I had a jam-packed day of errands and household tasks. It worked so well I could still recall everything . . . two weeks later. I had to mentally erase the images I had created in each of the rooms in order to use the technique again with another set of tasks and errands.

It was my pumpkin bread that needed baking, by the way. I had mentally placed a delightfully delicious-looking loaf of pumpkin bread in room #5. I envisioned it being perfect—and it turned out that way.

Aha! There might be more here than just guaranteed remembering. Next time, I'll place a really difficult task in one of the rooms and envision it going extraordinarily well . . . like hanging outdoor holiday lights. How about tangle-free cords and a tall ladder with mechanical arms that string the lights on my command? Now there's an image worth remembering.

CHECK. LIST.

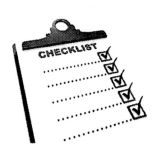

I am a list maker. In our household, we have two multi-itemed lists (one is taped on the pantry wall and the other on the back door going into the garage so it will not be missed). One is titled "Groceries," and today it includes soy milk, mangos, and dog bones. The other announces "Weekend Yard Work" and divides the pending tasks. There are notably more items in my husband's column. I like it that way.

I have a thoughtfully categorized list embedded in my iPhone. It acts as a reminder for daily tasks. And, yes, I occasionally put something that has already been completed on my list just to have the satisfaction of checking it off as accomplished. In checklist lingo, that's a "do confirm" action.

I am unapologetic about my penchant for making lists. Lists can change the world. You'll become a believer, too, after you read Atul Gawande's *The Checklist Manifesto: How to Get Things Right*. The author is a physician, so the book is a series of well-written stories about the effective (life-saving) use of checklists in surgery settings and clinics. One list starts with the simple reminder to "wash hands with soap." When this type of checklist was used in one hospital, the proportion of people not receiving appropriate care dropped from seventy to four percent. The occurrence of pneumonia fell by one-fourth, and twenty-one percent fewer people died as compared to the preceding year. Let's take time out here for a quiet, "Wow."

A riveting story launches Gawande's book. It's about a 200-pound man who got into an altercation at a Halloween costume party. The stab wound in his abdomen seemed relatively minor and the emergency room triage team did not think he was in immediate peril. Had there been a checklist requiring them to ask about the type of weapon that had caused the injury, their treatment decisions would have been quite different. In this case, it was a bayonet, which can cause a much deeper and life-threatening wound to the intestines. The guy survived—barely.

I want any hospital I'm in to use checklists—apparently ninety percent of physicians queried feel the same way. Checklists are not just used in lowering infection rates and saving lives in medicals settings, they're used in remarkable ways on construction sites. They are even starting to play a role in investment banking decisions. Of course, checklists are used in airplane cockpits.

Do you recall "The Miracle on the Hudson," when a US Airways jet was struck by a huge flock of Canadian geese right after take-off? The plane immediately lost both engines and was forced to land in the icy Hudson River. The pilot, Sully Sullenberger, and his first officer, Jeffrey Skiles, were highly experienced. The entire crew had a combined 150 years of flight experience and absolutely no record of accidents. It was a routine flight. It would have been easy for them to begin the flight without attending fully to the required checklists. But before they even started the engines, they ran through their checklists as a team—with practiced discipline.

So when the incident occurred, what do you think they referred to immediately? I am fairly sure it was their checklists.

PLASTIC BRAINS?

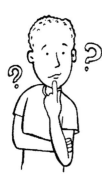 Think of your brain as "plastic." This is the word used by Dr. Kathleen Taylor, a professor at St. Mary's College in California, to describe thinking power in the aging brain. Dr. Taylor believes we all have the potential for more mental complexity and better recall abilities in our later years. She suggests that aging adults do not maximize their full mental potential, and we can easily improve our memory ability later in life if we become more self-challenging. Her exact phrase is, "Crack the cognitive egg and scramble it up." Don't you just love her way with words?

Studies indicate that if we want to sustain mental clarity throughout life, from midlife on, we need to work at "juggling our synapses." This can be accomplished by considering ideas and thoughts that are contrary to our own. Take what you believe to be true, and look at it from a new angle. Keep wondering about it. In the process you will become more mentally agile.

In a Sunday *New York Times* Education Life article published years ago, Dr Taylor and various memory experts talked about "How to Train the Aging Brain" or as I like to say, "How do we stay mentally clear to the end of our days?" The key seems to be to shake it up a little. What follows is my version of an example used in the article.

Let's say you have always believed Thomas Jefferson was a strong and admirable founding father. When asked, you call up his name with vivid examples of accomplishment. But what if you dug a little deeper into Jefferson's life and happened upon all those children he had with his slave, or what if you already knew about the children but you had never realized Jefferson was an abysmally poor public speaker?

Take something you strongly believe in and examine your knowledge base unrelentingly. Hang around with people who see the world differently than you do, and participate in friendly give-and-take conversations with them.

Sometimes it's as simple as doing something you do every day, but doing it differently. If you always hold your fork in your right hand, eat tomorrow's lunch with a fork in your left hand. Do you always take the same route home? Try another route. Floss in the morning? Start doing it at night. This is overall the better approach, by the way, so you might not want to switch back on this one.

The used-to-be-theory was that a huge percentage of brain cells were lost as we age. This has been found to be hogwash (not a term found in research, but accurate). It's quite the opposite; if we push ourselves mentally, the connections in our brains (the synapses) strengthen, grow, and multiply. Stretching our brains is what keeps them well tuned.

Is there any chance you don't buy my ideas on this? Maybe that's why you put a hot pad in the refrigerator yesterday and forgot your sister's birthday. Just wondering.

OUR GREATEST FEAR

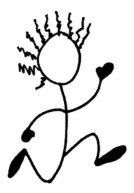

The greatest fear of aging for many of us is wrapped inside thoughts about losing our mental faculties. As one eighty-year-old woman said to me, "I'm fearful I might be losing my mind. I'd rather die."

If we are given the choice of dropping dead of a heart attack or stroke, versus languishing in a nursing care facility with Alzheimer's disease, most of us would choose the heart attack. There's reportedly research that says it takes a person an average of ten milliseconds to make this kind of decision.

But wait. Studies done at the Mayo Clinic indicate that specific health and lifestyle behaviors can help us avoid *both* cardiac problems and dementia. The evidence indicates that keeping a lid on blood pressure, blood sugar, and weight is important to more than just the avoidance of heart attacks and strokes. What's grabbing attention is new information that says regularly monitoring blood pressure, keeping blood sugar in check if you are diabetic, and maintaining a reasonable weight can also be important in averting the dementia that is called "Alzheimer's disease."

The possibility of losing one's mind is a tremendously big deal—even thinking about it can be unsettling. If you're a caregiver for someone who already has a diagnosis involving some form of dementia, you understand this a lot better than I do.

The cause of Alzheimer's disease remains unknown. So anytime there's new understanding or new ideas, it gets my attention. Research reported in the newsletter from the Center for Science in the Public Interest suggested that Alzheimer's disease and vascular dementia might be triggered by some of the same risk factors that result in other life-threatening conditions.

A healthy diet and regular exercise can help both the body and the brain—what a finding. One expert, Columbia University's Jose Luchsinger, put it well when he said, "It's a no-risk strategy; healthy weight, exercise, and a balanced diet are likely to be important for cognitive disorders . . . [but] the benefits are so large that if all you do is cut your risk of heart attack, stroke, and diabetes . . . there's no downside."

Here's more food for thought. We know that increasing the fruits and vegetables we eat, adding more whole grains, together with fewer soft drinks, less bacon and sausage, and perhaps a total abstinence from hot dogs is the wise way to eat. But it's hard to count carrots and opt for an apple when that bratwurst with all the trappings is calling to us.

Maybe with summer coming, a hot dog will look less inviting if we know that eating it not only increases our risk of heart and brain attacks (strokes), it also paves the way toward cognitive decline.

It's our greatest fear, so maybe it's also our best motivator.

SIX

ENGAGING SADNESS

I feel thin, sort of stretched, like butter
scraped over too much bread.
—J.R.R. Tolkien

Touch Me
Where Am I?
Depressed?
A Little Cranky Lately?
Doc Talk
Worried About Anything?
Selectively Happy
Pet Therapy
Does Prayer Heal?

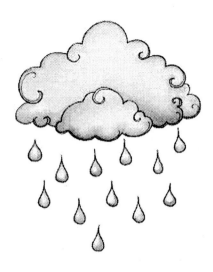

TOUCH ME

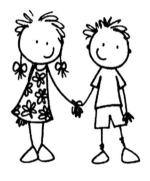 Did you know that if a teacher touches a student on the back or arm, the student is more likely to participate in class? And that the more athletes high-five or hug their teammates, the better their game? Did you know a touch can make patients *like* their doctors more? Maybe you were totally aware of this already. It came as something of a surprise to me.

The specific examples above were offered as part of a public radio program on a weekend morning. I've been pondering (almost obsessively) the power inherent in the simple act of touching another person ever since.

Let's try an experiment. This week, perhaps we can do two things. First, let's be more observant of the moments when one person is touching another. You know, those times when a small child reaches up to hold a parent's hand or a husband puts his arm around his wife as they sit talking with friends. Just watching it happen will probably be good for our collective spirits. These are challenging times and we need to draw comfort in all possible ways.

The second stage of this experiment might provide even more comfort. After you've done a bit of tender-moment observation, dive in and give it a try yourself. Dr. Tiffany Field, the Director of the Touch Research Institute at the University of Miami, describes it as activating the pressure receptors in the skin. Once engaged, through the simple act of touching someone's arm, hand, or back, these receptors send immediate signals to the nerve bundles deep in the brain, which then emit messages to the rest of the body, resulting in a slowed heart rate and a decrease in blood pressure.

A researcher at DePauw University describes it like this, "Touch buffers the physiological consequences" of a stressful moment.

I vividly recall preparing to speak before a large group at a national conference a few years ago. As I sat waiting to be introduced, the projector made a sizzling sound and the screen I had depended on to display my presentation went totally blank. I had a stomach-sinking reaction as I envisioned trying to be informative, let alone entertaining, for one solid hour without my colorful slides. At that moment, an elderly woman, who was standing nearby ready to introduce me, reached over and squeezed my arm. She did not say a word. There was no "Poor dear, such a problem this presents for you." She just touched me, and I will be forever grateful to her, whoever she is, for that brief, empowering physical exchange.

Some of you might be thinking, *I wouldn't necessarily want just anyone randomly touching me.* Okay—I can understand that. Maybe you could just perform the observational part of my proposed experiment. Be especially observant of mother and child moments. As I keep pondering all this, it occurs to me that moms (of any age) know the most about the healing power of touch.

Finally, if you're really not inclined to reach out and touch others more frequently, maybe the next time you greet someone you could just shake hands with a little more enthusiasm.

WHERE AM I?

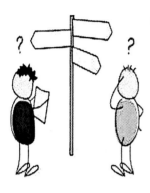

"I have lost myself." These were the words of Auguste D. in 1901. At age fifty-one, she became the first person to be diagnosed with Alzheimer's disease. Now it's a likely diagnosis for more than thirty-two percent of people over age eighty-five. Even as I type the percentage, I want to double-check it yet again . . . can it really be true? The thought gives me an uneasy feeling in my stomach.

The reality of living in our times is that huge numbers of people will be diagnosed with Alzheimer's disease over the next several decades. It's an epidemic, and we should pay more attention to it for many reasons—but most importantly because we are all living longer and because Alzheimer's is a family-wrenching condition without a cure.

For the individual with the diagnosis, memories fade away; some say they're "ripped away." Incoming thoughts evaporate. It starts gradually and proceeds slowly, with the time from diagnosis to death frequently reported to be between 8 and 20 years.

It's a disease that introduces personality changes and, ultimately, significant physical dependency. Loved ones turn into strangers. Some years ago, a public television broadcast "The Forgetting" profiled several families trying to cope with Alzheimer's. It's a sobering documentary to watch and it made me feel sad, but also strangely energized.

The documentary prompted me to ask, *What works? Is there anything that makes this incurable disease easier to manage?* Perhaps the answer lies in the fact that increasing attention is now being focused on the importance of early diagnosis and the prompt initiation of medications that slow the progress of the disease. We are also benefited because physicians know more about the disease than they did previously. In addition, the critical role of trained caregivers is better understood, as is the importance of support groups for families.

There's something else: empathy. This is a disease in which the person with the diagnosis might not recognize loved ones, but that same person might still understand the underlying tone of a conversation. If the tone is negative, the situation can get worse. In these circumstances, anger begets anger. Frustration in caregivers means those receiving care are more likely to exhibit frustration.

I am told that family tensions easily ignite because the person with the disease always believes they are right, and "right" can quickly turn into irrational righteousness. What often follows is a tense and angry dialogue where an already difficult situation becomes almost impossible.

Here's an approach to consider. Picture this scenario. Let's say I'm leaving the house with my dear-to-me, eighty-seven-year-old uncle, who is experiencing mid-stage Alzheimer's, when he says, "There's a rooster on the roof." Repeatedly. Relentlessly. Instead of responding with, "Come on, Uncle Earl. How many times do I have to tell you, there is no rooster on the roof?" I reach into my empathetic self, insert a little light-heartedness into the moment, and say, "And he's a damn good-looking rooster, too, isn't he?" We laugh . . . and we both feel better. Definitely less lost.

DEPRESSED?

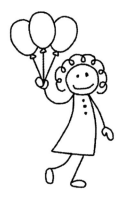

What do you do when you feel depressed? I have a set of ready-to-go, research-based coping approaches that can help improve a down-and-blue mood. Before I share them, let me offer this reminder. If depression is part of your life, please get professional help early. Depression is much easier to treat in its early stages; it can get worse and/or it is more likely to reoccur without treatment.

In the United States and worldwide, millions of people experience depression in some form. If this were any other illness, it would be a pandemic. Greater recognition of the broad scope of depressive illness is beginning to erase the stigma historically attached to this disease. Thankfully.

This brings me to yet another reminder. Depression is a medical condition. It is episodic and, most importantly, it is highly treatable. I consider www.mayoclinic.com a good resource for information.

If I feel flat and self-involved, which is my particular version of depressed (everybody's symptoms are different), I do one or more of the following:

I bask in the warmth of a sunny day. Sunscreen and a hat are advisable. For me, it's one of the best strategies for neutralizing down-in-the-dumps thinking. Try it. Find some sunshine and perch under it; contemplate something that is going right in your life.

If you're like me, you'll stay out there as long as you need to. Bring a friend, perhaps? If you feel like talking—do so, use the moment. Think of it as "letting the sad out." Supportive, listening family and friends are an incredibly important element in managing any form of depressive illness.

A sunny day is a particularly good thing if you have Seasonal Affective Disorder (SAD). This is depressive thinking brought on by seasonal realities. It's exacerbated by too many dark, wintry, confined-to-the-house days.

Physical activity and exercise absolutely improve mood, no matter what form of depression you might be experiencing. People diagnosed with depression benefit enormously from physical activity. For example, try a regular walking routine. I personally think thirty-five minutes is the magic number of minutes to walk on a daily basis, but you are welcome to increase the time and distance. Some folks say it's okay to "chunk it out" in ten minutes increments several times a day.

I'm not ignoring the severity and complexity of some depressions, but, for me, mild depression might be thought about in a way similar to the early signs of a cold. If I have a scratchy throat, I load up on Vitamin C and drink plenty of fluids. I get extra sleep.

If I start getting that flat feeling—I look to the ideas above, keeping in mind that early intervention is key. I might also think about whether I need to see a health professional to get my flatness thoroughly evaluated.

Irritability and hostility can be pivotal signals that depression is in play, particularly with older adults, in whom depression is more subtle. Other signs include ongoing complaints of aches and pains, and (this is a big one) memory difficulties. Memory difficulties masquerade as depression—and vice versa.

Now that you have a few coping approaches, hopefully it will only get a little sunnier from here on out. I am not trying to make this look easy. It isn't.

A LITTLE CRANKY LATELY?

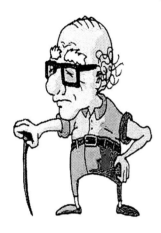 There is much to be said about crankiness and irritability as we age. The challenges that accompany aging are many; they can be incredibly unsettling. There's the issue of losing control (vision, hearing, and balance) or problems with digestion and constipation (the latter can be especially troubling). Maybe you get frustrated when you can't see the small print in a newspaper or on a restaurant menu. Maybe it involves hard-to-open plastic packages, or it irks you that your kids don't send thank you notes.

It's possible you were always a slightly grouchy person, and aging just accelerated your crankiness. No judgment here—but it's important to recognize this possibility and seek remedies. Another possibility: perhaps you've been happy-go-lucky throughout your life but someone died and you're in mourning. Irritability can be an indication of grief. It can also be a barometer for full-fledged depression. Excessive alcohol consumption might produce irritability; smoking cessation definitely makes people grumpy. My father did not drink or smoke (well, there was his evening pipe) but he was diabetic and his eruptive irritability was a definite reminder that his blood sugar was out of kilter.

For some people, irritability accompanies a diagnosis of mild cognitive impairment or dementia. Infections are also a big factor. Urinary tract infections (UTIs) can make an older adult confused, crabby, and out of sorts; sometimes the symptoms of UTIs resemble the symptoms of dementia.

There was a well-written article in *Men's Health* a few years ago titled, "Get Off My Lawn: Why Older Men Get So Grouchy." It was accompanied by a scowling, finger-wagging picture of Donald Trump, and it talked a lot about falling testosterone levels. I recalled that article when I was walking our dog last week and a man in a red truck drove by and yelled angrily, "Don't let that dog on my lawn." I waved my empty poop bag at him and smiled. But his outburst stayed in my head and led me to feeling glum. I think I snapped at my husband later that day.

Let's define irritability as "letting small things that happen in life set off a train of upsetting thoughts." I've discovered a simple way to constructively address this issue.

Start with self-assessment. Ask yourself, "How often do I get cranky?" Is it once a day or once a week? Pay attention to what sets it in motion (a spouse's scolding comment, a speeding driver who cuts you off in the parking lot?). Assign it meaning.

For example, did you get upset about the long line at the grocery store check-out because you were worried about getting everything done you needed to accomplish that day—or was it because you hadn't had lunch and your feet hurt? Once you've completed your self-assessment, think about what you could have done differently. Envision yourself doing it. Practice shifting your energy to something else entirely. Mentally walk away.

Then give yourself credit. You might even take your right hand and reach over and pat yourself on your left shoulder. Do it again.

DOC TALK

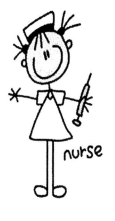
nurse

There are eleven things that we should talk to our health providers about. Maybe it's twelve. Different sources have different ideas about this. But they all say, "rank order the items" to make sure you cover the most important ones first. With a typical physician contact averaging around twenty minutes, planning what to say and making a list of discussion points in advance of your visit might be as important as the appointment itself.

A visit to your health provider can be difficult territory to navigate. First of all, when you show up in a doctor's office it's often because you're feeling poorly (or stressed and anxious) and unless you've thought about the discussion in advance, key areas might not get covered. Add to this the fact that health providers are often hurried or harried. They know they need to listen, but unless we make that easier for them, they'll go with the information they have available to them. One woman I know visits her physician with a prepared list in hand. She takes it out and begins to speak immediately after the health provider enters the room. She starts by saying, "Alright, I'm going to talk for three minutes. I'll watch the clock. Please don't interrupt me. I will listen to your reaction when I'm done."

The folks at Harvard suggest one of the things to talk about with your doctor is what you want to do, or used to do, but can't do any longer. Lab tests or a physical examination are not going to reveal compromises you've made. I know a lovely sixty-two-year-old woman whose sore knee prevents her from gardening, which has been her long-cherished pastime. The result is that over the last year she has had substantially less exercise with resulting weight gain, less sunshine, meaning less vitamin D, and a related bout with depression. If her doctor had known up front about the lifestyle changes resulting from her achy knee, doctor and patient working together might have been able to prevent some of her follow-along problems from her achy knee, doctor and patient working together might have been able to prevent some of her continuing problems.

If we do not tell our health providers about what we are afraid of, or where we have traveled lately, or even about another family member's recent diagnosis with a serious disease, they will not be as effective in dealing with our health and well-being.

Tell your doctor about all of the over-the-counter pills and supplements you take—and all the medications you have been prescribed by other doctors, and the medications you are supposed to take, but don't. Talk about your "personal stressors," smoking and/or drinking habits, and any incontinence or sexual dysfunction.

Choose the questions that seem the most important for you—the one regarding lifestyle changes and preferences really speaks to me, so they are at the top of my list. Personal stressors would be second.

Here is one more important tactic. Stay on message.

WORRIED ABOUT ANYTHING?

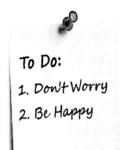

To Do:
1. Don't Worry
2. Be Happy

Worried about anything? Well, of course you are. There are always things in our lives that cause us concern. I'm quite anxious about a pending dental appointment and a little concerned about our dog's lethargy. Offer up the name of any of our three children and I'll easily identify something specific to worry about, probably more than one "something."

People have occasionally said to me, "You worry too much." Do I? When I hear this comment, I get defensive, and then I worry about being defensive. My best response when people say something like this is, "Worry is natural—a little normal anxiety is healthy." Worry encourages me to plan ahead, to be prepared. If I'm worrying about something, I'm thinking about it thoughtfully and creatively.

But if worry is a constant, nagging part of every day, it's not natural and definitely not healthy. There's even a name for this kind of worry, General Anxiety Disorder (GAD). I've concluded that I don't have a diagnosable anxiety disorder, but I've been worried enough about the possibility to do a little research.

This condition, according to the Anxiety Disorders Association of America, (which I didn't even know existed until I started worrying about worrying), is described as abnormal anxiety that's "irrational, intense, persistent, and out of proportion to any real threat." It's an excessive, uncontrollable, escalating concern about things that deserve to be worried about (a root canal) and things that don't (a napping dog).

Over four million people each year are formally diagnosed with anxiety disorders; the majority are women. GAD is a particular problem for women because it's frequently overlooked or misdiagnosed.

Health providers often think anxieties are a normal part of the "change of life" or a companion to complaints about aging in general.

Some experts say chronic anxiety in older adults is "grossly under-estimated" and important to reconsider, because if anxiety goes untreated there will be an increased vulnerability to depression or a full-blown panic disorder. In addition, people with anxiety disorders don't eat, exercise, or sleep properly, so they end up with fewer coping mechanisms when they are exposed to bacteria or viruses. If you ignore an anxiety disorder, chronic diseases can become more likely.

It starts with a friend's observation such as "You worry too much." But it's more involved than that. Symptoms include restlessness, extreme fatigue, difficulty concentrating, irritability, and muscle tension. It's very telling that over eighty percent of people diagnosed with anxiety disorders initially saw their doctors because of a physical complaint.

There are treatments and medications, of course. These days it seems like there's always a medication. But there are also some non-drug treatments that work quite well. Consider approaches like deep breathing, progressive relaxation, biofeedback, and cognitive therapy. Lifestyle changes can help, too.

Lately, when I feel worries coming on, I take a few deep, cleansing breaths. I also have another approach. I join our stretching-and-yawning-in-the-sunlight, hardly-ever-anxious dog . . . for a little nap.

SELECTIVELY HAPPY

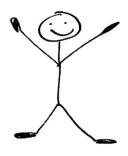 It seems old people are happier than their younger counterparts. I've just finished reading one of the well-researched articles in *Families in Later Life: Connections and Transitions*. This book is a compilation of studies and stories, many of which conclude older is happier.

So now you know. You can go ahead and keep aging, recognizing your social-emotional self will roll along a path of increasingly greater contentment. We are older and happier—but also, quite probably, less socially active. This is also supported by research.

Wait a minute. I always thought we needed social connections in order to be happy. I thought (maybe you did, too) that close relationships with family, friends, and neighbors were critically important aspects of aging optimally. Yes . . . but.

Here's the researched reality. There's undisputed evidence that our overall rate of social interaction declines as we age (most significantly, after we reach age eighty). We have far fewer direct contacts with family and friends—adult children are the exception, apparently—and we are less likely to volunteer or become members of a community organization. We are, in fact, more selective about what we want to do and, frankly, whom we want to do it with—even whom we want to talk to.

Lack of social connections can certainly lead to loneliness and depression and all sorts of undesirable outcomes. But there is another way of looking at this.

For some, social networks might be as large as always, but we are in contact with its members less often. This is just fine with many happily aging elders, or so it seems. Perhaps as aging adults we enjoy the anticipation of a contact as much, or even more, than the actual contact. Think about that.

Older adults who were interviewed for these studies indicated they felt like their days "were numbered" and they needed to make more "careful choices about expenditures of time and energy." One of the considerations used to make these choices was "Is this new information? Is this something or someone I really need to know?"

We are "old" after all, and we have heard a lot of this stuff before, so unless it's something novel or fresh we might just decide to pass.

As we age, we assess cost and benefit in coming to decisions about initiating or maintaining social contacts. We weigh the possibility (researchers say "the risk") of negative impact and act accordingly. As we age, we want to invest in the things that give us the information we need, as well as a positive emotional outcome. We are happy, after all. We want to stay that way.

PET THERAPY

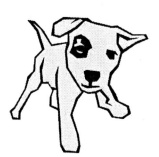

My friend Avalon lives with a parrot. We have a spaniel and a few of our neighbors have dogs or cats. The health benefits of pets, especially if you're categorized as an "older adult," are substantial.

Let's assume you like animals and you have a couple. Could it be that canines or cats, fish or ferrets are a part of your household? It's hard for me to envision ferrets making a positive difference in anyone's life, but maybe I'm underexposed. Whatever your pet preference, research suggests regular encounters keep you healthier.

A study done at the State University of New York at Buffalo found that people with pets have lower heart and blood pressure rates. One researcher with a definite sense of humor refers to it as the power of "pawsitive thinking." This is a little too cute for my taste, but you get the idea.

Pet therapy is common sense supported by science. The antics of animals at play keep you light-hearted. The presence of a dog prompts the daily walk you might otherwise postpone. Having a cat means regular exposure to contented purring, with its almost guaranteed-to-be-calming effect on your psyche. Furry critters encourage life-critical social interactions; feeding and grooming routines offer structure and purpose to a life lived alone.

But, as one of the pioneers of pet-facilitated therapy, Dr. Erica Friedman, puts it "pets are not medicine" and "although the presence of a pet has been shown to have a positive effect on heart rate and blood pressure, it's not clear that you have to actually own the animal to get the effect."

Staying with that train of thought, there are other issues to consider. Owning a pet can be expensive—and limiting. What do you do with your ferret when you go into the hospital for knee surgery? What do you do with an aquarium full of tropical fish when you take a three-week road trip?

For some, owning pets can actually promote negative interactions. A neighborhood cat's behaviors drive you crazy and your dog's barking drives your neighbors in the same direction. Science meets common sense, with a twist.

As you might have noticed, I am ever ready with solutions. How about this idea? If you already own a dog, walk it regularly and tell people who are so inclined that it's okay to caress your dog at will. If you have neither ferret nor parrot, or any four-legged pet in your life for that matter, look for brief encounters, with the accompanying therapeutic benefits.

Think about it this way. Feeding and observing a traveling neighbor's aquarium full of fish is a thoughtful, even healthful thing to do. Offering to house a neighbor's parrot for four weeks is a bit too much, but one day of parrot-watching might be possible. As for brief encounters with ferrets, I leave that up to you.

For my part, I have a loving spaniel who never barks. When I walk her, if we meet, you are welcome to pet her endlessly.

DOES PRAYER HEAL?

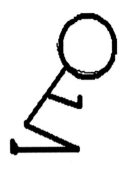

Prayer heals. If you have always believed this is true, you'll be interested to know that science might determine whether you're correct. In a Columbia University study of South Korean women undergoing in vitro fertilization, those who prayed were *twice as likely* to become pregnant. The study design was later found to be flawed. And there is research from the Mayo Clinic that concludes prayer on behalf of cardiac patients had no statistically significant impact on medical outcome.

Science seems increasingly more interested in ascertaining exactly what happens when prayer is a component of medical treatment. Research focusing on the power of prayer has nearly doubled over time. Previously anecdotal reports have been replaced by systematic investigations. The National Institute of Health (NIH) reportedly funded a four-year study investigating the use of prayer with women who had been diagnosed with breast cancer. This alone is an indication that things are changing. I am told that a few years prior, NIH refused to even review a study that contained the word "prayer,"

This we do know, *participatory prayer* (saying the rosary or chanting) can lower stress and blood pressure. *Intercessory prayer* (praying for others) is more difficult for science to examine. A study that would be truly fascinating is one where none of the patients would know other people are praying for them. Maybe they would not even know they were part of a study on prayer. Can you imagine how the medical community might come to attention, wide-eyed, if there were clinical findings that women with breast cancer who were prayed for by other women were later found to have significantly better health outcomes?

Many scientists question the appropriateness of addressing religious or spiritual issues in a medical setting. And yet people keep praying. It has been reported that ninety-six percent of hospital patients acknowledge using prayer as part of recovery. It seems to me if patients believe in the potential for a source of healing to such a degree, doctors would want to know as much as possible about what's going on and why.

Mitchell Krucoff, a cardiovascular specialist at Duke University and a proponent of the benefits of prayer, suggests that prayer "should not be seen as alternative to angioplasty," but instead be recognized as "the human being's need for something more, something spiritual that actually makes all the high tech scientific stuff work better."

While we await more scientific attention to this topic, you might want to do your own personal exploration of the healing effects of prayer. Perhaps we should offer up a collective prayer for greater world-settling and less tumult and political division.

Forever and ever. Amen.

SEVEN

FOOD MATTERS

A healthy outside starts from the inside.
—Robert Urich

Portion Creep
Popcorn Guilt
Spice Chaos
Lemon Heaven
French Eating
Tasteful Aging
Hot and Steamy
Sugar High
Mangos for Me

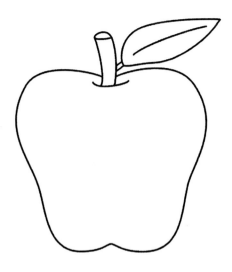

PORTION CREEP

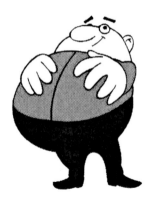

Have you heard of "portion creep?" It starts with a reminder of the Surgeon General's sobering statement, "Over sixty percent of adults are overweight." Or maybe it's more by now—that was last week. I did my own very unscientific sample, which involved the observation of people walking down the street one day. Every other person was visibly hefty. There were lots of big tummies spilling over too-tight belts.

The quite-large, older man with the 32-ounce Slurpee seemed to be enjoying himself. I wonder if he recalls the time when a standard size cola came in an eight-ounce bottle that contained 93 calories. The serving size he was indulging in has a total of 373 calories. I looked it up.

One couple I saw, both of them portly, was readying to eat bulging burritos. I wonder if they realized that a beef burrito with beans, rice, sour cream, and guacamole contains 1,640 calories. This is more than the number of calories that many women should eat in an entire day.

The same day I did my on-the hoof survey, my husband and I went out for an evening dinner at a restaurant. There were a lot of rich pastas on the menu. We had not one, but two, breadbaskets on our table with beckoning cups of parsley butter tucked inside. I ate several slices of the warm bread, a personal downfall, before my entrée, mushroom fettuccine, even arrived. You know that awful, too-full and mad-at-yourself feeling you get after eating too much? I hate that feeling.

Staying trim and enjoying accompanying health benefits is largely about self-discipline. But the reality is that there is really no plan where you can eat all you want and lose weight. You know that—it's a reality that is just a little hard to swallow. But there are tricks and techniques that help you eat more wisely in a world where food is often presented in larger quantities that anyone needs.

I asked a registered dietitian who maintains a consulting practice in my community about all this. She eats a lot, yet manages to stay slim and willowy. She had some very direct answers. Her recommendations are the ones I am going to follow. "Go to restaurants that have broad menus and healthy options. Order a la carte or choose an appetizer as your main dish. Don't hesitate to ask about the ingredients in a particular dish or how foods are prepared. Make special requests like the omission of salt or clearly state your preference for broiled meat instead of fried."

The advice goes on. At a breakfast eat-out, ask for fruit as a replacement for hash browns and, in the evening, request extra vegetables instead of pasta or potatoes with your meat. Stay away from the fettuccine altogether.

And if we ever eat out together, please *don't* pass me the bread.

POPCORN GUILT

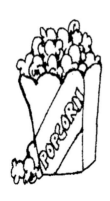

Here's the scene. It's Friday at the end of a long week and my husband is out of town. I'm yearning for a night out, so my friend (let's call her "Nancy") and I seek an early movie. And we decide it's a "popcorn for dinner" night. Ever done that? It's quite freeing.

We arrive at the theater and walk to the concession counter to place our order, going way overboard with the size of the bags and the amount of butter. So far I'm just anticipatory—not feeling guilty at all. After all popcorn is a whole grain food and we actually need fat in our diets on a daily basis. (I did not make that up.)

As Nancy and I turn away from the counter, I see two friends in line for the same movie—and they see me. They observe our big bags of popcorn and our hands dipping in. So, of course, they shake their heads. Big grins light up their faces, fingers are wagging—was there actual laughter? Now I do feel guilty.

You probably know the reason; the story originally surfaced many years ago. The Center for Science in the Public Interest published a report condemning "Movie Popcorn." The movie theaters included in the report were found to be selling popcorn popped in coconut oil, which was later dredged in a butter-margarine combination. A small bag reportedly had 29 grams of not-good-for-you fat. For the record, that's approximately equivalent to a breakfast of bacon and eggs, a lunch consisting of a Big Mac and fries, and a steak dinner. (I didn't make this up either . . . sigh.)

I remember feeling very sad when that report came out, and for a while I took to making and eating my popcorn at home and not in theaters. It was a much smaller screen and far less butter. But this particular movie night was more than a decade later and the popcorn-damming report sort of slid out of my mind. I've had other things to think about —and after all it was a Friday night after a long week and it's a whole grain food (or did I already tell you that?).

I think it's important to set the record straight. Popcorn can be an excellent food option. If it's air-popped, no additives, one cup contains relatively few calories, loads of fiber and even some protein. It's a friendly food. I favor big puffy butterfly-like "flakes" with good mouth feel. (I'm getting hungry just writing this.)

It's the powerful aroma that attracts me the most. You too? Or maybe it's the fact that there's no other way to eat it but with your hands. Did you know that popcorn is the official snack food of the State of Illinois? Does your state even have an official snack food? You might want to look into that.

I favor popping my corn in a kettle over the stove using a constant shaking approach; it raises expectation and serves as a little exercise before I dig in. Bet you never considered that.

How about looking at it like this. Considering every other possible indulgence, occasionally eating movie theater popcorn does not even seem indulgent. Maybe next time I'll have a smaller bag . . . maybe.

SPICE CHAOS

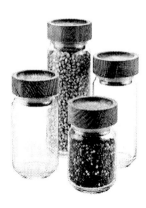

Have you ever unexpectedly found something, some out-of-the-blue piece of information that captivated you totally?

For example, quite by happenstance, I learned several of my neighbors alphabetize their spice shelves. I was incredulous. I would never have thought about doing that. Then I wondered if a lot of people did it and maybe I'm just not in the loop.

I kept thinking about this. I gave a community presentation a few days later and decided to ask whether anyone in the audience put their spices in alphabetical rows. (The topic I was speaking about was not in any way related to my question, but I thought I would just use the moment.) Hands raised in response to the query indicated one-third (maybe more) of these women (and a few men) did exactly that.

I stand in awe, completely. At this moment, I'm perched in front of our overflowing spice cupboard and have issued a challenge to myself. Find the turmeric in less than thirty seconds. I used it to make tofu look more like scrambled eggs just yesterday morning, so I'm thinking it's probably near the front. Looking . . . looking.

New challenge, I'm going to try again. Find the nutmeg. I use it to flavor meats—it reduces my tendency to over-salt and I think I read somewhere it might have a positive effect on the cardiovascular system. I'm still looking. There it is. How did the nutmeg get way up there on the top shelf next to the coriander? Now that I'm rummaging around, I better pull that citrusy coriander closer to the front. With Thanksgiving coming, I'll need it to give texture to my sauces.

Did you know that coriander is actually cilantro, a source of dietary fiber? Who would have thought?

I should look for the cumin, too. If I were an alphabetizer, it would be fairly straightforward right about now. I need cumin for my winter-friendly turkey chili, which calls for a whole tablespoon. Cumin is a somewhat underrated spice, I think. It gives foods such a rich and toasty flavor.

I digress, but I do want to share that cumin is being studied for a possible connection to cholesterol reduction. Spice aficionados already believe it aids digestion. It's probably a good thing there's so much of it in that bean-filled chili. Speaking of chili—I just located the red chili peppers. I would never want to misplace that bottle. Studies suggest chili peppers are associated with everything from pain relief to stomach ulcer prevention.

So here I am standing on a sturdy stool in front of our chaotic spice cupboard realizing change is in order. I'm also coming to understand my spice shelves are a lot like our family's medicine cabinet and I need to treat them with more respect.

Okay, everything out, check expiration dates, toss (i.e., recycle bottles) as needed, wipe off the shelves and the remaining bottles. Start anew. Maybe I will even find attractive glass bottles that I can label myself.

Let's begin with anise. Like many of the examples above, it's actually an herb and reportedly helps manage stress, which I'll probably have less of after I've completed this alphabetizing task.

It could take a while—but I'm worth it.

LEMON HEAVEN

For much of my adult life, I have been trying to perfect lemon meringue pie. I envision a crust that is melt-in-your-mouth flaky with a velvety, tart, lemon zest filling. I see myself creating a lemon pie where the first forkful prompts a sigh of complete satisfaction, perhaps even a faint, indulgent moan. Lemon heaven.

I have found my pie-making approaches to be quite popular. Friends and neighbors are more than willing to do taste tests. My husband hopes I never "get it right," so that I will keep trying.

I use a 100-year-old recipe called "Lemon Pie Supreme" taken from a church cookbook that has been in our family for decades. It calls for fresh eggs and grated lemon peel. It's the kind of pie that was probably cooled in a farmhouse window while a warm summer breeze wafted gingham curtains past a lightly browned meringue.

That's what this message is all about—more the cooling and less the pie. This is a food safety lesson masquerading as a lemon meringue pie recipe. It is a message targeted at older (aging) adults.

As we age, our immune systems become more vulnerable. Less-than-fresh eggs can sometimes make you ill . . . that would be eggs that take too long getting from the laying chicken to the cooler, or that have been stored in your refrigerator for more than two weeks. Farm eggs that are not washed well, or even a lemon that's not thoroughly cleaned before grating, can wreak havoc with our immune systems.

A lemon meringue pie allowed to "cool" in the warm sun, or remain out of the refrigerator for more than two hours, has the potential to produce food borne illness in anyone. For an elderly person, the resulting illness can be much more than just nausea or stomach cramps; it can be life-threatening. Older adults are more at risk, and once they become ill, it takes them longer to recover.

Food borne illnesses (there are hundreds of different varieties) are caused by pathogens (bacteria). Typically, these annoying little bacteria grow and multiply on hot food that is not kept hot enough or cold food that is not kept cool enough. These bacteria thrive in moist, high-protein environments—like that lemon supreme pie with its three beaten egg yolks and two tablespoons of butter.

I plan to keep trying to perfect my lemon meringue pie and testing it on all ages, including precious elders. I will wash my hands before preparing it, and I will wash the eggs before I crack them and the lemons before I grate them.

My luscious pie will cool in the refrigerator—unless, of course, it's eaten immediately after it comes out of the oven.

FRENCH EATING

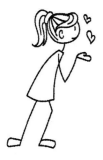

When asked to respond to the words "chocolate cake," Americans say "guilt" and the French say "celebration." I just finished eating a dish of Chocolate Brownie Thunder ice cream (two scoops). It was melt-in-your-mouth good, with huge chunks of rich, fudgy chocolate throughout.

And yes, I'm feeling a little guilty. But I enjoyed it enormously. I ate it slowly and savored each delicious spoonful. It took me almost twenty minutes and the last creamy taste actually made me feel a little sad. Celebration over.

In Mireille Guiliano's book *French Women Don't Get Fat*, we're reminded that we don't take enough time with our food. The thin and lovely author tells us to linger over meals, enjoy food more. She would probably encourage my Chocolate Brownie Thunder moment, but would suggest I use the "good china" and eat each spoonful even more slowly than I did (one celebratory scoop only).

This is the other issue—it's not about what you eat, but how much. In a French restaurant you might get sauces but you won't get super-sizes. According to a University of Pennsylvania study, American portions are twenty-four percent larger than other cultures. We eat more and we eat it faster. The average amount of time it takes to eat a fast food meal in France is reportedly 22.2 minutes. In the U.S. it takes 14.4 minutes. That stated, why anyone would opt for McDonald's or Burger King when eating in Paris, I do not know.

How fast we eat and how much we pile on our plates is important information to have. For example, I do better when I recognize that my protein source (meat, seafood, tofu, or nuts) should be about the size of the palm of my hand. Now, if you're a small person with very big hands, this rule might not follow, but for most of us it's a good gauge.

The parameters are five to nine servings of fruits and vegetables each day, which means 2 cups of fruit and 2 1/2 cups of vegetables. My dietitian friends say keep a twenty-four-hour food journal and see how you do—then do better.

In France, eating is pleasurable and it's done differently. It's always an experience. French adults eat at three fixed meal times. They rarely snack. Their children might snack after school, but adults defer. Becoming a little hungry between meals is seen as entirely appropriate. Foods speak to them, but in a more beautifully disciplined fashion.

We all have foods that speak to us. Other than the beckoning thought of rich chocolate ice cream, my biggest food-related hurdle is that I absolutely love avocados. Unfortunately, the recommended serving size is 1/8 of an avocado. Ouch.

Madame Guiliano would suggest I eat that avocado, just not eat one every day. And slice it quite thinly. She would encourage the use of a small fork and suggest I place the avocado in a little glass dish lined with fresh spinach—and add fresh pepper and lemon. Oooh la la.

TASTEFUL AGING

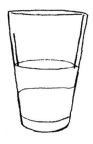 Did you know our taste buds change as we age? After age forty, the number of taste buds we have starts to shrink, i.e., "lose mass vital to their operation" as some experts explain it. After age sixty, we can lose our ability to differentiate the taste of sweet, salty, sour, and bitter foods.

I was skeptical the first time I heard this. Ever innovative, I tried an in-home test. I was fairly sure there would be no change in my ability to identify the salty taste of a dill pickle or recognize the sour taste of a lemon. It was convenient that these two foods happened to be in our refrigerator. The dill pickles were in the back of the second shelf from the top behind the mustard. They were a bit on the dated side, so they were not the best choice for this totally off-the-cuff exploration. The lemons were plump, bright yellow, and just-purchased.

I cleansed my palate with a large glass of water. Then I focused thoughtfully and recalled the best taste I had ever experienced eating a crunchy dill pickle in terms of saltiness. I remembered the moment well. It was a picnic decades ago; there were lots of big, fat, salty pickles. I ate several. On a scale of 1 – 10, the salty taste I recalled was a definite 10. I tasted my just-found pickle and made my assessment on that same 1 – 10 scale. The saltiness of the pickle was nowhere close to my original recall. Have you ever wanted to sprinkle table salt on a dill pickle? That was my reaction.

Continuing my taste test, I recalled my first experience with lemons. A diet plan I launched decades ago was my introduction to using lemon juice instead of salad dressing. The juice of a just-squeezed lemon and a little sea salt sprinkled on a bowl of arugula can be delicious. But I realized half a lemon had become an entire lemon. I quickly recognized I was now using greater amounts of lemon juice on my salads to get the remembered taste, and I also realized that I was adding more sea salt.

Changes in the perceived taste of foods might explain why some older adults gain weight. We keep eating more food in the hope something will taste like it used to taste. Ironically, it might also explain why many older adults lose weight. To them, nothing tastes good anymore.

There are other things to consider about a changed sense of taste; over-salting foods or over-eating salty foods can lead to hypertension and related health problems.

If this gets your attention and you want "tastier aging," or if salt consumption is an issue in your life, I have a few ideas. Did you know that basil and cardamom are good salt substitutes? Grating the peel of a lemon or lime to create a zest before you squeeze out the juice on that bowl of greens is another approach. Try finely chopped ginger, and think about using more minced or powdered garlic.

We have choices in everything we do. These are the relatively simple ones.

HOT AND STEAMY

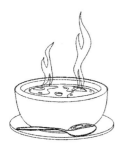 At certain times of the year, a bowl of hot, steamy oatmeal can be the ultimate breakfast pleasure. My version includes a few added raisins or walnuts, some low-fat milk, and a teaspoon or so of sugar, preferably brown. Even *thinking* about oatmeal for breakfast makes me feel like I'm taking better care of myself.

When I was growing up in southern Minnesota we called it "porridge." It was not oatmeal, but cream-of-wheat-with-dates. I had this delicious bowl of hot cereal almost every morning, usually accompanied by toasted Wonder Bread, freshly squeezed orange juice, and the comic section of the newspaper.

Cream of wheat is well-remembered, but I would like to make a case for oatmeal becoming the hot and healthy breakfast of champions for older adults. The array of health benefits it offers is staggering. First of all it's a high fiber food, which means it keeps us regular. As people age, regularity and the potential for constipation can become a preoccupation. Might as well get any concerns about this addressed and out of the way first thing in the morning.

There's more. Oatmeal also has a research-based impact on chronic disease. It definitely reduces cholesterol. In fact, it was the very first food product allowed to make a formal health claim. This means the Quaker Oats folk can announce the benefits of reduced heart disease right on the oatmeal package. If you're diabetic, oatmeal helps maintain blood glucose levels. If you have high blood pressure, it can have a measurable impact on lowering it. One study found that individuals who ate three servings of oatmeal (11.68 grams of oat fiber) a day could reduce or even eliminate their blood pressure medications.

I'm not formally recommending that much oatmeal in a given day, although you might think about this reality. If you had a large bowl of oatmeal for breakfast, snacked midday on yogurt with added oatmeal and blended a little oatmeal into your dinnertime turkey burgers, you could actually pull it off. If you choose to do that, embrace the idea gradually.

We should not over-eat anything, and definitely not modify a cholesterol-lowering medication regimen without consulting a health provider. That said, this kind of research so wonderfully reinforces my hot and steamy breakfast of champions point. I simply had to include it.

Supposedly eighty percent of American households have oatmeal in their cupboards. Old-fashioned (rolled) oats is what I recall, but now we seem to opt for something more quickly made. The Quaker Oats products are the ones most of us remember. As an added benefit, those lovely, big round containers the oatmeal comes in have so many uses, once they are empty.

When my daughter was small, they were perfect for storing the tiny hard-plastic toys we seemed to constantly step on. I made an oatmeal-box "purse" that doubled as a drum for my granddaughters. However, it did not work out so well when they tried to turn it into a chair.

My preferred steel-cut oatmeal takes a fair amount of time to cook, just long enough to let the dog out, scan the headlines in the morning newspaper and check out a few comic strips.

Worth waiting for—a healthy, comfort food, at any age.

SUGAR HIGH

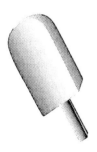

It's a gloriously sunny, spring afternoon and a girls' softball tournament is underway. Families have come to watch the games and cheer for their teenage daughters and sisters. A concession stand fills the air with the smell of chili dogs and warm nachos. You can sense the expectation—anything could happen.

My attentions are focused on an attractive, but weary-looking mom and her husky blue-eyed youngster. The boy is what some might call "a handful." He's a sturdy tyke who's constantly on the move. His attention span can be measured in seconds. This big-for-his-age four-year-old seems to ask for and get pretty much whatever he wants. By the third inning of the first game, he has eaten two rainbow ice pops, two small candy bars, one large bowl of startlingly blue ice cream, and a "bubbly."

When he asks for it by name, I think he means the kind of bubbles that you buy at the dollar store and blow out slowly through a handheld wire hoop. Nope, his quickly-downed "bubbly" is a brand name soft drink that, by my calculation, has over 70 grams of sugar in a 24-ounce cup.

You can envision what happens next. There's a public meltdown. It's a hard-to-watch, out-of-control tantrum that makes parents and grandparents squirm with embarrassment. Attention to the playing field is diverted by the sideshow. It's a screaming, thrusting, ground-thumping few minutes with "I want more ice cream!" as background music.

I could be wrong, but I believe this incident is all about the high sugar content of things like rainbow ice pops. I'm bolstered in my assessment by a newspaper article titled, "Is Sugar Toxic?" by Gary Taubes, who also wrote *Why We Get Fat*. The author takes a compelling look at sugar consumption and discusses the work of Robert Lustig, the leading expert on childhood obesity at the University of California, San Francisco School of Medicine.

If the softball field scene resonates with you in any way, and you have children (or grandchildren) with defiant behaviors, or if your own sugar consumption is not entirely defensible, this kind of information is worth reading. It won't improve your knowing how to reduce sugar intake in nearby four-year-olds, but it might make you think twice about what you eat for lunch.

The Food and Drug Administration (FDA) estimates that we consume 40 pounds of sugar per person per year beyond what we naturally get in fruits and vegetables. The United States Department of Agriculture (USDA) is usually thought to have the more reliable data in this area and they estimate 75 pounds per person per year. No wonder one in every three Americans is considered obese and diabetes is so prevalent.

Some researchers believe sugar is "poison." A Colorado State University study found that if you feed animals enough fructose (sugar), their livers convert the fructose into fat, the kind that supposedly causes heart disease. Changes can happen in as little as a week if the animals are fed sugar or fructose in large amounts (sixty to seventy percent of their diet). Stop feeding them sugar and the fatty liver promptly goes away. The research is not conclusive but it is compelling. It goes way beyond the "empty calories" argument. And if you throw in a public tantrum or two, it gets even more interesting.

As one researcher puts it, "Sugar scares me . . . officially I'm not supposed to worry because the evidence isn't conclusive, but I do." Yup, me too.

MANGOS FOR ME

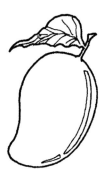

When the morning paper arrives, my husband goes out to our driveway wearing his too-big robe and raggedy slippers and picks it up off the pavement. He trudges back into the kitchen and starts to read it, standing by the counter with a strong cup of French roast coffee in his hand. He begins by scanning the front page. Then he moves to the sports section.

Finally he turns to the "Healthy Living" section (surely he will turn). And when he sees my column, he begins to read it. After a few moments, he glances over at me, and giving me a look as though he can hardly believe it, he says, "Your column is on . . . mangos?"

I usually ask this husband of mine to read each of my weekly newspaper columns before I submit them, but over the past week he's been traveling a lot and was not really available. Truth be told, I expected he would question the wisdom of my creating an entire 520-word essay on mangos, so I deferred on making any before-the-fact announcements.

I look over at my husband, who I do not think has ever eaten a slice of mango in any form because he is a Granny-Smith-apple-and-banana kind of guy. I suspect he is, in fact, cringing a bit right now at the very thought. Hang on . . . dear. Ready yourself for something deliciously grand.

My affection for mangos began when I had my first few succulent slices earlier this week. Oh my! How could I have lived for sixty-plus years without the delight one gets from a slice of juicy-dripping-rich mango?

Eating a mango makes me rethink fruit in general. I am serious about this. Once I found them and they found me, I started thinking about mangos constantly. They rolled into my mind immediately upon waking in the morning every day this week—really. I bought three of them at the Co-op and gave one to a neighbor, and then immediately regretted it. I wished I had kept all three. It's almost an addiction.

Their nutritional value is more impressive than almost any fruit I've encountered. Lots of fiber and antioxidant-rich vitamins A, C, and E. There's even some calcium. As an added benefit, mangos smell heavenly—to me, it's an aroma reminiscent of lilies of the valley and freshly mown grass.

I prefer mine ripe and raw, but mangos can be turned into fruit preserves of all kinds including lovely chutneys. Several folks tell me grilling mango slices with poultry in some form is even better than eating them fresh. I shall assuredly try that. In some cultures, less ripe mangos are eaten with lime and salt—or on a stick with a little chili powder. I might try that, too.

It's still Tuesday morning. I have a breakfast surprise for my now smiling (but only slightly) husband. I've completely peeled a ripened mango and cut across it at one end to create a flat bottom. Then I sliced large, checkerboard chunks almost down to the flat, fibrous seed at the center. It fans out in a really attractive and come-hither manner. Shall we indulge, dear?

There is a little part of me that wants him to remain unenthusiastic. That way, there will be more for me.

EIGHT

FAMILY FACTS AND FABLES

When your mother asks, "Do you want a piece of advice?" it's a mere formality. It doesn't matter if you answer yes or no. You're going to get it anyway.
—Erma Bombeck

Alex and the Unexpected Super Heroes
Shopping with Sydney
Toby—A Uniquely Grand Dog
Sarah Gets Taller
Love, Jordan
Big-Hearted Rose
Remembering Being Hooked
Connection
Love and Marriage

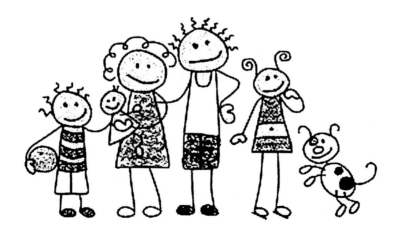

ALEX AND THE UNEXPECTED SUPER HEROES

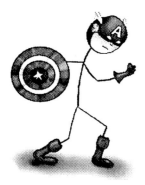

If you spend a Christmas holiday with your grand-children, there might be a movie involved. For us, it was an afternoon at a cinema near Charlotte, South Carolina with our six-year-old grandson, Alex. I recall him as beside himself with joy in anticipation of this outing. I was fairly excited, too. Time with a child is its own gift, and the movie was unexpectedly engaging.

It was a lively two-hour animation titled *Rise of the Guardians* depicting the collaboration between Santa Claus, the Easter Bunny, the Sandman, the Tooth Fairy, and Jack Frost—with the goal of saving the world. Working together, they proved to be incredibly effective.

Jack Frost was a little icy about the possibilities at first, but he ended up being the overall hero, although everyone involved deserves some credit. It was all about give and take among independent entities, each with very specific agendas. Success seemed based upon forging mutuality around a common mission, i.e., preserving the wonder and well-being of children. I kept thinking throughout that there were lessons in this movie for our country's elected leaders. Actually, there were loads of messages.

Our grandson sat between us eating popcorn, one butter popped kernel at a time, eyes riveted on the big screen. At one point, he leaned over and whispered in my ear, "I didn't know the sandman had so much power!" as he watched a glittery sand-ball put the boogie-man-bad-guy into a deep sleep. My husband was already sleeping, so I think he missed that part.

I remained wide-awake throughout, reading into every action or reaction a message of some kind. I always over-think things when I go to the cinema. For example, Santa appeared unexpectedly Russian and he had a large, ornate tattoo on each forearm that read "naughty" (right arm) and "nice" (left arm). Or was it the other way around? You got the impression the Russian Santa did not tolerate much "naughty."

The Tooth Fairy, in case you have been wondering, was absolutely delightful. She resembled a hummingbird, and smiling baby hummings fluttered around her constantly. As the female lead, she was fearless. I liked that. The Easter Bunny was fearless in a different way. He was definitely not soft and cuddly, but rather a tall, scruffy-looking, aging rabbit with an Australian accent and an attitude. The message resonated. He seemed like a reminder that we might have some unexpected surprises as we age.

All of the childhood fantasy characters in the movie were portrayed a little differently than one might imagine, and I must admit it made me a bit uncomfortable. But, as you know, these are challenging times and it's probably good that we, as parents and grandparents, get outside of our comfort zones sometimes. It will make us more vigilant over the long haul.

"If you believe in good things, bad things don't happen as much," said Alex when the movie was over. This is such a great sentiment. Let's make it work.

SHOPPING WITH SYDNEY

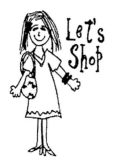

You might not believe this, but it's true. Dr. Marilyn Albert, a prominent memory expert, researcher, and professor of neurology, has determined that shopping is good for the brain.

In 1985, she and her researcher-husband began a ten-year study of 3,000 older adults. They found three things that are important for memory to work optimally in the aging adult:

1. Stay physically active.
2. Challenge your brain to constantly make decisions.
3. Maintain a positive self-image.

Sounds like shopping to me.

I tested the concept by spending a morning and part of an afternoon at our local shopping mall with our soon-to-be-college-freshman granddaughter.

I remember it well. This lovely young woman is quite athletic and known for being the pinch runner on her high school softball team, so we stayed on the move for five hours and thirty-two minutes. I did not count the number of stores we went into, but a dozen sounds about right. By the time we reached the last one, we were also doing a certain amount of strength training because of the weight of the packages we were carrying.

Every store we entered challenged my brain. There was the ever-present pounding musical beat and impossible-to-identify songs. I actually tried, at first. The racks of densely-packed clothes were set up like mazes, and once you entered it became apparent the only way out was through the cash register.

"Grandma, what do you think of this?" The first time Sydney said this, I was tempted to respond with "Don't you think it's awfully short and a little "see-through?" But I didn't have to say it, because after just a few moments of contemplation she herself observed, "I don't think my mom would approve." Let it be noted, I felt a deep, brain-cleansing sigh of relief and admiration for both of them at that moment.

It was a mind-challenging shopping adventure, in part, because our eighteen-year-old granddaughter was such a tiny little thing. I had never been shopping with someone who tried on clothes that were size two! In fact, I didn't realize there were so many stores in our local mall that had clothes in that size. Some of them were merely pieces of fabric so small that it seemed they should be given away for free—like napkins in restaurants.

My brain exercised itself as I tried to keep the intended budget in my head. The options for purchase and the big word, SALE, pulled and pushed us toward endless offerings of clothing that Sydney suggested would be "great for long nights at the library" or "perfect for studying in my dorm room." Sydney plans to enter a nursing program, but I really think she has a future in marketing.

But let's go back to the third point in Dr. Albert's original research findings. "Shopping enhances self-image." In this case, I did not even have to test it with purchases. It was indisputably affirmed when one store clerk smiled at me warmly and said, "Such a composed and lovely granddaughter you have . . . ." Yes, I agreed, I do.

TOBY—A UNIQUELY GRAND DOG

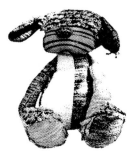 Our rescue dog, Toby, was a long-haired terrier mix, originally part of a Humane Society project that retrieved soon-to-be-put-down dogs and found them new homes in other states. Our neighbor at the time was a veterinarian at the local Humane Society. She knew I had a heart as big as Canada and she needed a favor.

Let me paint the picture of this dog's beginnings. Toby was a particularly challenging placement. He weighed next to nothing and had a nasty puncture wound on his right foot. The record indicated his previous owners had actually nailed his foot to the floor. I know—it's hard to even write this for you to read.

His medical issues were further complicated by a treatment-resistant case of pneumonia and an unwillingness to eat. And there was another consideration; he barked in a shrill, uncompromising way whenever he was left alone for even a few minutes.

It was a difficult first couple of months. But finally Toby began to eat and gain weight, his wound healed, and he recovered from pneumonia. After some trial and error, his barking was reasonably well controlled by using a "bark collar" that emitted citronella spray whenever he even breathed heavily. He only wore it a few times. Fairly quickly, all we had to say was "Bark collar?" and the barking ceased. However, the whole house continued to smell like Citronella for months.

Toby was defined by coarse, bristly hair that stuck out at all angles. When our daughter saw him for the first time, she said, "Can't we get him some conditioner?" At just about that moment (as I recall it was the same introductory visit), he looked up at her for a mournful moment, walked over to me, lifted his leg high, and peed on my shoe. I think he was offended by her remark. Or maybe he was jealous and claiming me because he was afraid I loved my child more than him.

Toby had an array of idiosyncrasies. Yes, they were directly related to our (make that "my") enabling behavior. When he finally decided to eat again, Toby preferred a seven-inch glass plate placed just to the left of his water bowl and rotated once while he was eating. He liked little lumps of one particular kind of moist dog food positioned around the edges, a few pieces of kibble, and just a sprinkling of Mexican cheese on the top. And carrots, he loved raw carrots. He had to have them offered one at a time—baby carrots, not too big.

These were all manageable issues. Toby's only really enduring problem was his continuing reluctance to walk on wooden floors—which we had a lot of in our home at that time. He would tiptoe a short distance across a wooden expanse, but only if there was a particularly tasty carrot awaiting him. Even then, it took cajoling. At one point, I put a series of paper towels down on the floor and created a path to his food bowl. My husband wisely pointed out that moving the food bowl to a new location was the better strategy.

Here is the application to aging. Have you ever been in an assisted living facility or a nursing home and witnessed the joy that results from even a brief visit with any kind of dog. Dogs are a common connection to the past—to family and children and grandchildren, and a less complicated time. One sage person once said, "Dogs are forever young . . . they remind us to love unconditionally despite the pressures of the day and the burdens of age."

Toby is no longer with us—but we salute him. He dug his little feisty self into our hearts.

SARAH GETS TALLER

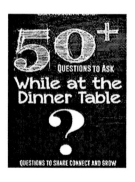

My husband has a penchant for asking questions that prompt engaged discussion. He's often able to pose provocative, probing queries and encourage those around him to consider something in a fresh way. Here's the scene. We're having a family dinner, everyone has indulged maximally, and dessert is about to be served.

My spouse introduces the idea of a question-sponsored discussion, and before the people at the table can disagree, he starts it with, "What are your seldom-stated goals for the next year?" Our eleven-year-old granddaughter, Sarah, responds right away, "I know this isn't very deep, but I just want to be taller than my sister." You go girl! Her fourteen-year-old sister displays an indulgent grimace and then offers up her desire to become a photojournalist. She states her intention to take steps in that direction over the coming months. At least that's how I remember it. Who knew?

The rest of the family expresses goals and objectives that center on improving health or achieving a personal best. But Sarah's honesty gets the most thoughtful and reflective follow-along discussion.

What if the questioning moved to: "How are you going to change the world?" Some people find this question off-putting. My husband asked that question once and a dinner table guest, a recent retiree from the health field, acted mildly affronted, saying, "I spent my career trying to change the world! I rather resent the idea that I'm expected to keep trying when I just want to relax and read books that are on the Sunday *New York Times* best seller list."

That, not surprisingly, leads to a discussion about the *New York Times* Book Review, and more specifically a regular feature titled, "By the Book." In a past issue, the person interviewed was Margaret Atwood, who has written fascinating books over many decades. Her newest contribution is, *The Heart Goes Last.* One of the questions posed to her in the *Times* Book Review article was, "Tell us about your favorite fairy tale."

This kind of question usually generates discussion at our dinner table about how *Power Ranger and Avenger* videos have replaced *The Collected Work of the Brothers Grimm.* It can lead to an eye-opening conversation on the changing role of media or the increasing availability of wearable technology.

In his book *A More Beautiful Question: The Power of Inquiry to Spark Breakthrough Ideas*, Warren Berger argues, "We are all hungry for better answers, but first we must learn to ask the right questions." My curious husband with his inquiring mind would be pleased to know Berger believes, "Creative, successful people tend to be expert questioners. They have mastered the art of inquiry, raising questions no one else is asking and finding answers everyone else is seeking."

I believe beautiful, well-stated questions stage the possibility for change; they make us think—more completely, more deeply. Perhaps instead of taking what we hear, which might or might not be evidence-based, we reflect on a fact or a related idea more thoroughly, turn it over in our minds, and analyze it through conversation. In the process, we can become more informed about possibilities we have not previously considered. It's the kind of thing that makes us taller.

LOVE, JORDAN

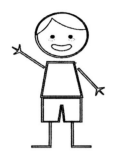

Here's the scene. It's a birthday party for my two-year-old grandson. There are nineteen toddlers scampering around inside an enclosure of huge, inflated play structures. Other family members are busy hosting the celebration and I've been designated to watch the Birthday Boy.

Wearing a superhero T-shirt and a wide grin, he beckons me to follow him as he heads toward a wheezing, heaving apparatus near the back of the room. He crawls inside. I see no option but to follow, while trying to suppress my trepidation. We slip inelegantly on the bouncy surface and rock onto our knees. I feel neither safe nor in control, but I'm spurred on by my grand-boy's infectious giggle. Another series of openings loom, and they seem even narrower than the first. I squeeze my ever-widening derrière through one of them. It's way too dark inside and we are, once again, rolling and bouncing in all directions. I catch a glimpse of rubbery, protruding steps up a slippery-looking incline.

My grandson leads the way; I hesitate because I'm not sure I'll be able to make the awkward climb. And then it happens. My two-year-old grandson reaches out his pudgy little hand to help me. No words, just a smile and a hand to hold. Panting just a little (that would be me, not him) we emerge at the top of the structure, see the slide, and go down it together. It was a lovely moment I will remember forever. Have you had one of those lately?

The power of hand-touching-hand is vividly present in a video-gone-viral that displays sea otters in the Vancouver Aquarium floating around on their backs "holding hands." With them, it's not just cute; it's a natural instinct called "rafting" that keeps the otters from floating away from each other in rough waters. See the parallels here?

A University of Wisconsin study found that hand-holding reduces feelings of fear, loneliness, and physical pain. Apparently the more positive you feel about the person whose hand you're holding, the more powerful the impact. Ponder your own experience with this. Don't you think there's almost always an unexpected easing of stress and tension from the simple act of touching? Not just hand-holding, but also a gentle pat on the arm, perhaps? Maybe it's a handshake, but one that exudes warmth and caring. I mentioned this in an earlier chapter—see how important it is. It gets an encore.

Think about how this might apply to your own life. Yes, it can be risky. Some people are touch-adverse. I think they just need more practice. Children do it best and most naturally, reaching out for a hand or a hug, snuggling onto a shoulder for comfort. Perhaps you could start like this. Identify some children in your life—inflatable play structures optional; hang around them more often. Let them lead the way.

BIG-HEARTED ROSE

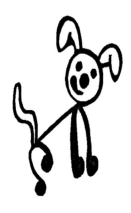

I once spent a Sunday afternoon in a darkened theater clutching a soggy wad of tissues. Like millions of dog-lovers, I was succumbing to the draw of "Marley and Me," the movie about a yellow lab who wreaks havoc on a household. I didn't realize an afternoon at the movies would generate such a combination of laughing and weeping. Anyone who's owned a chew-at-random dog can probably relate.

My husband once had a lab that dug up every inch of his back yard. Every single inch—and it was apparently a big yard. After we married, our dog of choice was a Basset Hound. In retrospect I'm not sure why—it was the long velvety ears and soulful eyes, I guess. In her first week with us, Maxine chewed the arm completely off a piece of furniture.

Now, you're probably thinking, "How can people allow that to happen; weren't they watching that dog?" Yes, we were; but she was quick—and we were eating dinner at the time. And, yes, I'm still just a little defensive because it was supposed to be *my* day to watch the dog. I'm not entirely sure whose day it was when Maxine ate the dog training video. We'd rented it. The folks at the pet store laughed so hard when we returned it to them (as a gob of mangled plastic) they didn't even charge us.

When our family relocated at a distance, we felt it was time to find an adoptive home for Maxine. We did, a family with four small children. A card the following Christmas indicated Maxine was doing well. All the children were intact, although apparently their stuffed toys had been disappearing at a fairly rapid rate.

We've had other dogs through our thirty years of marriage. The most memorable might be big-hearted Rose. We acquired her on a cold, blustery February day. It was the day of my beloved father-in-law's funeral.

It seems a little strange to have made that particular decision on such a day. In retrospect, we should have named her "Herbert" in his honor.

But she came with the name "Rose." She was a brown and white Cavalier King Charles Spaniel born at the exact moment the Trade Towers fell. We acquired her from a breeder who had been raising dogs for a long time.

The most recent litter had been large and Rose was the last to be placed. She was reportedly flown across country in an airplane cargo hold. But her new owners decided they didn't want her after all, so back she went. Just for us, is how I saw it. We were in love from the moment we saw her big brown eyes and silky soft fur.

Our Rose was the kind of dog that made people smile, Other than exposing her belly to complete strangers in order to get a quick tummy-rub, she really had no bad habits. No barking of any kind, no jumping up on people coming to the front door. Sweet temperament—although she did eat my reading glasses—but the optician said he saw that a lot.

Her best trick was napping. She did that really well. We calculated that one day she slept over twenty hours. This should have been a clue, I guess.

At a relatively early age, Rose was diagnosed with life-threatening cardiomyopathy (an enlarged heart), hence the term "big-hearted Rose." We are fortunate that my sister is a veterinarian and our neighbor at the time was a veterinarian who made house calls, and the new medications for canine cardiac conditions worked extremely well. Until they didn't.

I think about Rose a lot. It's true you know . . . that saying, "I want to become the kind of person my dog already thinks I am." Ever trying.

REMEMBERING BEING HOOKED

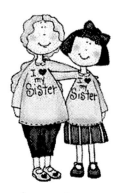

Many summers ago, we spent the better part of a long weekend with two of our very-young-at-the time grandchildren. We had sunny, frolic-filled afternoons at a local spray park, several hard-to-go-to-sleep bedtimes and countless loud, lusty sing-a-longs. There were messy eating experiences involving large quantities of Cheerios and multiple glasses of chocolate milk. Oh, and we had hotdogs with massive amounts of ketchup.

I can hear you—you're reading this and saying, "Do you know what they put in hot dogs? You fed your granddaughters hot dogs?" Yes, I did. Twice, in fact.

I have several insights about that particular grandchild-for-the-weekend visit. And it goes beyond regret regarding the hot dog issue. By the way, several dietitians I know say it doesn't really matter what you feed a child, just so you eat while sitting down around a table together, talking about your day and life in general.

I was then, and am still, completely hooked on being a grandparent. The rewards are countless—big and small. I recall that precious moment during our visit to a toy store, when I heard, "I'm glad mommies don't look like Barbies." On hearing this, I emitted a small hallelujah! Out loud.

There had been an earlier, before-the-visit indication from my daughter-in-law, who has always known and understood her children extremely well, that there were are only seven kinds of food that Bella liked. But when Bella visited us for that weekend, she ate a whole container of peach yogurt for lunch one day—so then there were eight.

Perhaps this was what riveted me to this special time. Maybe it was Bella's sage observation during a contemplative moment, "When I'm nice, people like me more." I think the most common sense remark

---

How Gray is My Valley

came from both girls—it occurred during an evening dog-walk, when we heard, in reaction to a STOP sign, "Anytime you see one, don't go."

"Don't go." That's how I felt when they left early on the final morning. Our two youngest granddaughters, Bella and little Sarah, lived at such a distance they did not visit as often as we might prefer. When they did, it was bliss (well, most of the time). When they left it was sad (always).

There are so many obligations and responsibilities involved in raising a child. I am extraordinarily admiring of young families today. When these girls were young, my daughter-in-law managed two active children solo for days at a time because our son, a pilot, was flying. When he came home, he assumed the parenting while she stepped solidly into her passion as a classroom teacher. I salute them. They have always been extraordinary parents, bias acknowledged.

Family situations change over time. Ours certainly has. These two girls are now in their teens. Visits like the one depicted above don't happen much anymore. This is why I like to tell their early-on stories. Someday when they are all grown up, maybe a small child will say to them, "Grandma, tell me a story about when you were little." And they will be ready.

CONNECTION

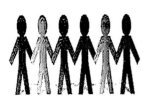I recall learning about an epidemiological study initiated after the World Trade Center tragedy. A year after September 11, 2001, a team of researchers sought out and interviewed people who were living in the immediate proximity of the Twin Towers. These individuals had experienced horrific trauma resulting from the events of that day, in some cases experiencing significant losses and permanent physical disabilities. The research team wanted to find out who coped well in this type of situation—and why. They hypothesized it might be older adults or more educated individuals who handled the aftermath more successfully—possibly women rather than men.

This is what they found. The people who managed themselves the most optimally in all facets of their lives were the ones who had strong social networks—a collection of readily available, caring people (family, friends, and acquaintances) who would listen thoughtfully, allowing these survivors to share feelings and "get the sad out."

Having recently spent a lovely weekend with close friends, my husband and I returned refreshed and renewed, feeling more relaxed and connected with each other than we had in some time. I think I understand what happened.

We talked a lot. We discussed communication challenges, shared affections, and how to problem-solve. Our friends told us stories about what worked (and didn't) during their forty years of marriage. We learned about ourselves by hearing about them. And in the process we laughed often and more heartily than usual. We left our concerns behind and indulged in what I now think of as a social rejuvenation.

There is an incredible power in friendship. My desire to know more is prompted by a book, *The Blackberry Tea Club: Women in their Glory Years.* It's a book about many things, but largely about how family and friends sustain a woman in her fifth decade who is experiencing loneliness and personal challenge.

There's a place in the book where the author (Barbara Herrick) raises the question that Oprah Winfrey (friend to all of us) originally asked. "What do you know for sure?" There are the obvious answers: "This body is the only one I'll have," "Our children deserve our best selves," and "Anything can happen at any time." We also know that "Laughter is as necessary as bread," "What is loved, loves back," and "We can't do it alone, whatever *it* is."

We can't do it alone. Research is highly supportive of social networks as a significant component in over-all well-being. The Nurses' Health Study, sponsored by the Harvard Medical School, found a woman's social interactions to be a significant predictor of freedom from bodily pain and increased vitality throughout the aging process.

I'd like to be pain-free and full of vitality well into my 90s, and it's nice to know that outcome doesn't necessarily have to come in pill form. Maybe I don't even need to increase the length of my morning walk. I'll just call up a friend and arrange to meet for a cup of tea.

LOVE AND MARRIAGE

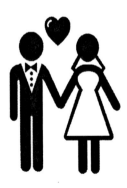

When you go through decades of married life as a blended family, awkward situations sometimes arise. If you're in the forty-two percent of people who have at least one step-relative and you have a wedding to plan, you know exactly what I'm talking about. One of the more incredibly stressful events of my life revolved around our daughter's wedding eight years ago. Her handsome fiancé was Hawaiian and the venue was . . . yup.

I should immediately clarify it's not really "our" daughter who got married; it was my daughter, actually. But she and her siblings, my husband's two children from his previous marriage, had lived with us since they were in middle school, and we always tried to refer to them as "our children." Well, not always; during those difficult later-adolescent years, there were times I didn't want to claim any of them.

In this daughter's case, she had waited a long time to get married and she had a vision. She also had layers of interested and excited "stepped family" relationships; her fiancé, whose parents were also divorced, had even more interesting stepped arrangements. In Hawaiian families, the aunties are like mothers and all the aunties wanted to come to the wedding. Maybe this is way too much information. It probably is, but I'm trying to tell a story here.

Family events like weddings require decisions. I am not referring to who gets invited. Of course, they all do. But where do they sit—especially if you have the wedding and reception in a venue with large round tables that each seat eight people?

As we got into the final planning moments, the biggest issue of this way-too-big wedding involved positioning people at tables. The intention was to position them in a way that did not create awkwardness, or even worse, insult. It was incredibly tricky.

Here's an example. The day before we flew to Hawaii for the wedding, our kitchen table was covered with large, colorful cardstock tents; there were equally colorful and flowery place cards with names on each. It was my daughter's preference to have guests identify their tables by matching photos of native Hawaiian flowers (of which there are a total of fourteen—and we had nineteen tables; but that's another story). And yes, I'm the mama who said— "Oh I can find exactly the right photographs and make all those tents and place cards. It will be fun."

Actually, in recollect, it was sort of fun—except that with all those parent-types (if you include godparents, there were a total of eleven) who started weighing in about their preferred seating arrangements, it quickly became challenging. I used a luncheon plate to draw nineteen round "tables" on a large piece of paper. As I was doing this, my husband, who was fixing dinner at the time (bless him), called out, "Have you seen the cover to the lemon pepper?" I laughed and said, "I'm using it in wedding preparation." And that might be the last time we laughed heartily at anything related to wedding planning until the actual day. Please don't misunderstand; it was truly wonderful. The Aloha spirit rolled over all of us. There was Hula dancing performed by one of the nieces and my grand new son-in-law serenaded the beautiful bride with ukulele music.

And I think, as often happens at weddings, a few grudges evaporated and one or two new alliances formed. I thought about putting my ex-husband (who was divorced, yet again) at the table with my new son-in-law's delightful and unmarried mother. But my daughter nixed that idea.

Just call me Cupid. Well, actually call me mother-of-the-bride. Wait, that was eight years ago. Just call me Nana.

NINE

GIVING CARE

Some days there won't be a song in your heart.
Sing anyway.
—Emory Austin

Gob Smacked
Find Another Mother
Living with the Kids
Poignant Kinship
Mothering Behaviors
Don't Kill Granny
The Story
Chortles and Snorts
Feeling Loved and Feeling Safe

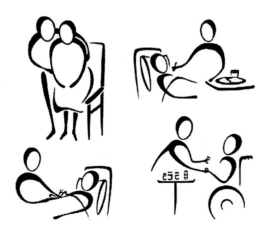

GOB SMACKED

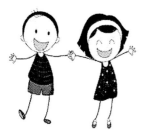

The term of the day is "gob smacked." As in, "I was gob smacked when my son asked me at what age I thought I might want to go into a nursing home." He really did say that, and if he is reading this right now . . . may I just suggest to my beloved stepson, keep reading.

The term combines the English/Scottish slang word "gob," which means mouth, with the verb "smack." If you're "gob smacked" you're totally astonished, solidly hit with something that leaves you speechless.

Recently I was wide-eyed and open-mouthed while reading *Independent for Life: Homes and Neighborhoods for an Aging America*. In each chapter, contributing authors illustrate the possibilities offered by creative, age-friendly thinking and new technology. Some of this information might prompt hand-to-an-open-mouth astonishment in you as well. Let's find out.

Envision it's a decade into the future and you're determined to continue to live independently, i.e., age-in-place. But your children are worried. Maybe you are, too. Here's one creative idea. Have a "shake sensor" installed on key objects in your home. The sensor non-intrusively tracks your normal routine. Do you get out of bed at a regular time, take your medications in a timely fashion, and get daily exercise? A sensor on a medication bottle or your walking shoes could inform you about unrealized changes in activities of daily living as well as assure information is transmitted to your adult children living at a distance. The unobtrusive device conveys a sense of "okayness" to concerned family members, or perhaps it raises a caution flag. It assuredly provides early identification of possible problems and prompts solution-oriented thinking. By the time you read this, sensor technology might have been replaced by something even better.

Here's another idea that might have a gob smacking effect on you. In neighborhoods and communities where folks of all ages drive their cars and some older adults are stuck at home, GPS units (global positioning devices) can be temporarily placed on the dashboards of neighbors' cars to determine typical routes (grocery store on Tuesday mornings, church on Sunday). This information could then be shared with stay-at-home seniors living in the same neighborhood and ultimately match willing drivers with those who need rides or errands run. The result would be more social connectedness for lonely aging adults and engagement across neighborhoods.

Here's why this kind of technology is so critical. Aging experts tell us there's "an epidemic of isolation among older people." It's well-documented that once an individual's social support system has declined, health inevitably fails. One study has already shown that continuous measurement of everyday functions such as walking, can detect changes that can indicate cognitive decline. Researchers found individuals with a rich social network are measurably healthier and live at least 1.6 years longer than their age peers.

Let's go back to the concept of in-home sensors as a further example of the unexpected impact to be realized when you have more information. In a study a few years ago, sponsored by Intel Corporation in concert with the Oregon Health Sciences University Center for Aging and Technology, sensors were placed on the telephones and entryways of a sample of aging adults. These sensors tracked calls and visitors to the home. Many of the adult children were gob smacked by the data collected. A typical incredulous reaction was, "Your system must be broken—the display says my father has not had a visitor or a phone call in six days!"

The system was working just fine.

FIND ANOTHER MOTHER

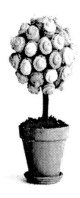

Imagine this. You're sitting in a room full of people who are attending a lecture. The presenter is a professor from Stanford University who has a doctorate in public health and an international reputation. She's talking about her research on individual and family health. Someone in the back of the room asks a question. It's long and rambling and involves the challenges of relating to and caring for an elderly, ailing mother.

The professor's response comes in a matter of fact manner and without hesitation, "Find another mother." There's a collective gasp in the room. (I was there; I know.) For a few moments, the entire audience sits in disquieted silence.

But the response makes perfect sense. Think about it. Think about the possibility of trading mothers for a little while. Perhaps you could give some of your caregiving challenges to another person and, just for a short time, assume theirs. You might identify a friend or neighbor who has an ailing mother and switch circumstances for a few days or weeks. The concept offers an admittedly unique respite (of sorts) as well as an opportunity for a fresh perspective on caregiving obligations.

The idea of "finding another mother" has stayed with me. Have you ever heard the phrase, "There's no reason to have the same thought more than once, unless you really like that thought." I really like this thought.

There might be other versions of this "find another mother" concept. My own mother died over a decade ago. It doesn't seem that long, but it is. And my godmother-aunt died several years later. I miss them, especially around holidays. Oh, I have kids and grandkids who will always need mothering and a spouse who requires his fair share.

But I have an excessive amount (overflowing actually) of motherly inclination. I need to have it in play somewhere.

So I am open to providing a little respite for someone who is drowning in caregiving responsibility. Maybe it's just one day or maybe it turns into a caring-over-time relationship. I like both versions. Much needed respite is a missing element for family caregivers. I'm thinking there might be a lot of "mothers for a day" before too long. Hallmark might even get on board.

LIVING WITH THE KIDS

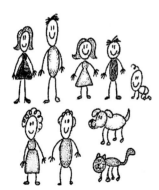

I recently received correspondence from a friend who was planning to relocate. It sounded like a move to be "closer to the kids." She was full of mixed emotions about it.

At the risk of sounding harsh, I reject the idea—not completely but almost. Let me begin by affirming that I admire all our children and their spouses, and all the progeny that have resulted from their unions. I even love the grand-dogs, except the pooch that ate my favorite leather shoe—him, not so much. But he left his small rubber toy in the gummed and mangled toe of my shoe and, I have to admit, it was rather endearing.

But let's stay on topic. Let me restate something. Permanently relocating in the immediate vicinity or in any of the homes of our adult children beckons me minimally. Quite probably, it beckons them minimally, too. I have really thought about this and even tested the concept. I can see living in the same city, but not close enough to drop in without calling first. Maybe we see this differently. Think about it.

Temporarily helping out during a baby's first year of life, or extended childcare while frustrated parents take a break—of course. Taking select grandchildren for an entire summer? I know that could work. Having our children or grandchildren move in with us temporarily if their financial situation required it? As necessary, I would assuredly do that.

But this I know. In preparation for the final decades of life, I want to do everything I can to live independently. I want to be in a place that my family looks forward to visiting. I am more likely to have this option available to me if I start planning early.

Whether you share my desire for independence or just want to assure the best possible living situation and/or be closer to your oldest daughter and her family, now is the time to think about how that might look and review the choices involved.

The website www.grandparents.com posed the question: "Should You Move Closer?" Three aging couples talk about their decisions, how they made them, and why. The site references an AARP survey that says eighty percent of grandparents want to be closer to their grandkids. If I had completed that survey, I would have been one of the respondents in the eighty percent category. I want to be closer. I just don't want to live next door on a forever-and-ever basis.

If you are contemplating a move, there are a few key questions to ask:

1. How difficult would it be to move in terms of lost friendships?
2. Do you make new friends easily?
3. Is your child or his/her spouse likely to experience job relocation in the near future?
4. Are they likely to make frequent moves, such as every two to three years?

Ask yourself lots of questions. Think through all the options. Research them. Make an informed choice and then embrace the decision you've made. Always embrace the decisions you make—until you cannot.

POIGNANT KINSHIP

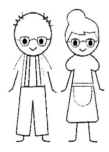 Some years ago, I spent much of a weekend day "watching" two of our young grandchildren. Did you know it's possible to hold a one-year-old on your right hip while using your left foot to assist a three-year-old on a tricycle roll up an incline? If you do it several times in a row, you get better at it.

I cared for two active children for a portion of just one day, and at the end of it, I was completely exhausted. I cannot imagine filling that role full-time. But many grandparents do. One local eighty-plus grandfather I know is parenting three grandchildren under age six. One grandmother with chronic health problems has parented a three-year-old since he was born.

According to recent census figures, there are tens of thousands of grandparents who parent full-time. These are aging adults who have already raised one family and are raising another. "Off Our Rockers" is the term one support group used to describe themselves.

Often the parenting involves a kinship component. An aging aunt takes in her deceased sister's teenagers; a widowed step-dad raises toddlers that are not even blood relatives. But it's grandparents who are the centerpiece of second-time-around parenting.

It can be sudden or slow. A long-unseen daughter arrives at your doorstep with a small child when you didn't even know you had a granddaughter. Or you're in the role of childcare provider and there comes a moment when, as one grandmother put it, "I'm no longer watching them; I'm raising them."

Grandparents have always served as support for their children and grandchildren. But what's happening right now seems different. Some data suggests one in twenty grandparents is fulfilling the role of full-time parent. The reasons are often referred to as the four "Ds," drugs, divorce, desertion, and death. Drugs and alcohol create eighty percent of the problem, by most reports.

The phrase, "I didn't need a child, but the child needed a mother" stays in my mind. There are other phrases that linger as well, like this one from *Grandparents as Parents: A Survival Guide for Raising a Second Family:*

> *I live with my grandma because my mom left me on a hotel bench to get a cup of coffee. You're not supposed to leave babies by theirselves.*
>
> —Erica, age 11

That's right. You're not supposed to abandon children, and "grand" parents don't. What a huge task it is for them, however, and what a toll it must take. Is this you—or someone you know? I hold you in my heart.

MOTHERING BEHAVIORS

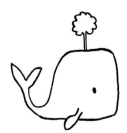

The well-known author and poet Alice Walker says it like this, "We are not over when we think we are."

The somewhat less well-known author, Lauren Kessler, says it differently in her book *Dancing with Rose:*

I cared for my mother on my own for exactly eighteen hours . . . we drove out to the airport to get her . . . she spent the night . . . hours later I dropped [her] off at a care facility . . . a clean, modern, trying-hard-not-to-be-institutional place with six vacant-eyed women sitting in the living room. I got out of there as fast as I could. When I got home I took the nightgown she had worn, the one I lent her, and put it in the trash. Just in case Alzheimer's was contagious.

Some experts say the best protection against landing in a nursing home is having a daughter. From my own experiences, I believe this to be true. However, I think having a niece helps, too. But this is not that kind of story. At least, not in its beginning.

This is the story of a daughter who was not equipped, not emotionally able, or simply not willing to provide the diaper-changing, bath-giving, spoon-feeding care her mother, who had mid and then late-stage dementia—more specifically stated, Alzheimer's Disease.

It's the story of that same daughter who, after her mother's death, sought peace (perhaps some would call it atonement) in a minimum wage, hands-on caregiving position in a locked memory-care facility. And in the end, something that seemed awful turned out to be quite beautiful.

The story begins like this. It's Lauren's second day on the job and she's feeding a patient who *. . . chews and chews and chews* *and chews . . . but doesn't swallow. She has forgotten that this is what you do when you have food in your mouth, that this is how you eat.* It is said Alzheimer's patients become like babies who have to be dressed and fed and toileted. There is some truth in this—except, as the author quickly reminds us, They are not babies. *Babies love your touch. Babies learn.*

After a few weeks into her job, Lauren starts to find her caregiving rhythm. But then, an accident occurs . . . inevitable, avoidable, unsettling, and very messy.

This book is incredibly direct. It's a gut-honest and unflinching look at Alzheimer's disease. It profiles consummate caring in one paragraph and digs into the raw, rich discussion of caring-barely-at-all in the next paragraph.

It casts tender light on the incredible load faced by caring families and paid caregivers. Not just for months or years, but throughout lifetimes. It talks about Alzheimer's disease and dementia in ways that wrench your heart (and maybe your stomach—sometimes both). It's sadly exquisite reading.

Perhaps you're saying to yourself, "This doesn't apply to me, I'm not a caregiver." You will be.

DON'T KILL GRANNY

It all started when an aged neighbor knocked on our door over a decade ago and handed me a photocopied newspaper article; he was unusually imperative. As I recall he said something like, "Read this . . . now." The headline was, "The Patients Doctor's Don't Know" authored by Dr. Rosanne M. Leipzig, a physician-professor at Mt. Sinai School of Medicine.

The second sentence said it all, "American Medical Schools require no training in geriatric medicine." I knew at the time there weren't many geriatric training expectations for graduating docs—but "none?"

I am hoping things have changed or are changing. But at that moment in time, and verified with a little additional research, all medical students were required to have experience in pediatrics and obstetrics, even though after they graduated it was noted they will probably never treat a child or deliver a baby. Geriatric training required: None. Did I say that already?

Does this make any sense? Say it with me—"no." Or as the doctor-author of the original article put it, "This shouldn't happen." And here's the real capper, over eight million in Medicare dollars each year goes into training medical residents. See why I'm so agitated? Deep breath . . . .

This means graduating doctors are less likely to understand that a seventy-year-old person with severe depression might present very different symptoms than a thirty-year-old person with a diagnosis of depression. For the record, in an aging person there are more physical-in-nature complaints. There are more aches and pains, and less sadness and moodiness.

There are loads of disease conditions that present themselves differently as we age. For example, bladder infections and the confusion that accompanies them can easily be misdiagnosed as dementia. A knowing doctor might understand the complex nature of urinary tract infections in aging adults, and there are those that do. But experience is likely to be their teacher.

I have found a few things that give me hope. A group of caring health providers, who are clearly aware of the exploding demographic of aging adults, developed something they refer to as the "Don't Kill Granny" list which contains reminders about such things as the importance of fall prevention discussions with older adults. I am not sure I have found the actual list (still looking) but I understand it includes reference to the often-unrecognized hazards of hospitalization for someone in their eighth decade.

There is some good news. An Institute of Medicine report about eight years ago titled "Retooling for an Aging America" discussed the issue comprehensively with recommendations. The stated goal went something like this: "The achievement of minimum basic competencies by medical students that assure quality of care for older adults." I take issue with the words "basic" and "minimum." But maybe that's just me. I sort of take issue with "quality of care," too. Perhaps we should be focusing on "quality of life."

I am heartened by well-told stories in Dr. Atul Gawande's incredible book, *Being Mortal; Medicine and What Matters in the End.* He talks about a geriatrician colleague whose goal is to bring "as much freedom from the ravages of disease as possible and enough function for active engagement in the world." Sounds like quality of life to me. Give your primary care physician a copy of *Being Mortal.* Read it first yourself—my graying and bespectacled friends. Highlight the phrases that speak to you.

THE STORY

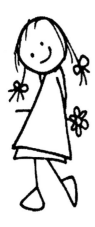

I'm about to tell you a story . . . backwards.

Once upon a time there was a nursing facility (some people refer to these environments as "post-hospital rehabilitation settings." Sometimes they're called "skilled nursing homes"). This particular facility was full of people who were ill or debilitated. Most were in their seventies and eighties, but not all. Some were, in fact, quite young.

Many were recovering from surgery, a heart attack, or a stroke. Pain medications filled the trays distributed by attentive nursing aides. Oxygen tubing was everywhere and catheter bags hung from the edges of beds. The residents needed assistance with bathing and eating. Only a few were able to toilet independently.

Remember . . . this is a backwards story, so I started at the end.

The beginning of the story might start with Doralee. She was a resident of this facility. Throughout her fifty-five years of living, Doralee smoked several packs of cigarettes each day. She stopped in her late forties, a few years before a diagnosis of lung cancer. She has always carried thirty pounds of extra weight and defended her years of smoking as a justification for not being even heavier. She admits she never paid much attention to what she ate. She preferred desserts to vegetables and ate "more coconut cake than carrots." When asked about regular exercise, Doralee said her achy, arthritic joints usually prevented her from moving around a lot. And yes, she knows that regular physical activity would probably have made those joints less achy but she "could somehow just never get started . . . ."

There's more to the story. Research has identified that people who adhere to all four of the most basic healthy behaviors remain the healthiest throughout their lives. These behaviors include:

1. Not smoking
2. Maintaining a healthy weight
3. Eating adequate fruits and vegetables, and
4. Exercising regularly

I cannot tell you where Doralee would be right now if she had never smoked and kept her weight adequately managed. I do not know if eating more vegetables would have kept her out of a nursing home, and I cannot do more than surmise what would be going on with Doralee if she had exercised daily. But I believe her story would have been much different.

The real story is this. Doralee is like all the rest of us. The actual percentage of people who observe all four of the above-identified healthy behaviors (as outlined in a 2006 issue of *Consumer Reports on Health*) is an unbelievable three percent.

Write your own story—make the ending happy.

CHORTLES AND SNORTS

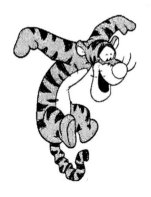

In case it's been a while since you experienced a joyous, all-consuming belly laugh, the kind that leaves you breathless and smiling out loud, I'm going to attempt to provide you with one. I draw from the advantage of having a four-year-old in residence for a week. For future reference, small children and puppies are almost guaranteed to produce random giggles and an occasional chuckling snort.

We did not have a puppy around this past week, but we did purchase two goldfish for our grand-boy. My husband thought we should name them "Melania" and "Donald" because "they seem a little fishy." But we went with Disney characters instead. The one who was completely orange we still called "Donald," last name Duck.

We specifically chose fish because at bedtime our grandson was afraid of "the bad guys coming." He describes them as "zombies, witches, cheetahs, tigers, and fish." I thought a bowl of cavorting goldfish might distract him and neutralize some of his fear. But he later informed me the only "really bad" fish are sharks.

I came up with what I thought was a rather brilliant way to eradicate all "the bad guys" by filling an empty spray bottle with water and marking it "Bad Guy Spray," specifically naming the culprits on the label and allowing him to spray wildly if he thought one was around. It actually worked well, although his pillows and pajamas got quite damp the first night. As a side benefit, "Jordan-boy," as we call him, can now spell "cheetah."

Laughter is usually defined as "rhythmic contractions of the diaphragm in response to internal or external stimuli." Done well, it can be quite aerobic. Elders who happily watch comedy show reruns on television instead of taking a walk around the block could use this as a defense if challenged about not getting enough exercise. Although some of both—daily physical activity and regularly enjoying chortling, guffawing, tittering, cackling, and sniggering is preferable.

An on-line article in *Psychology Today* a few years ago described laughter as "full-on collaboration between mind and body." It releases tension, lowers anxiety, boosts the immune system, and aids circulation. I must admit, the first time I read that article I almost went out and bought a puppy.

Another on-line article from *Psychology Today* was titled "20 Rules That Everyone Can Live By." The first rule was "Bring your sense of humor with you at all times. Bring your friends with a sense of humor. If their friends have a sense of humor, invite them, too. Remember this when going to hospitals, weight-loss centers, and funerals, as well as when going to work, coming home, waking up, and going to sleep."

I recall laughing around the supper table on the day of my dad's funeral. At the time, we were recalling when he almost set himself on fire in church after he put his still-lit pipe in his shirt pocket, and then interrupted the sermon trying to explain what had happened—with smoky tendrils curling around his head and the congregation doubled over in laughter.

Dad was in an unexpectedly competitive race for church council president at the time. And yes, he won.

FEELING LOVED AND FEELING SAFE

Thank you!

I have a vision that someday I will round up women in their eighties and nineties who are living alone in little houses and apartments without any connection to friends or family, and I'll invite them to lunch. There are so many of them, it might end up being several lunches. I will serve an airy quiche and colorful little fruit cups. There will be a dessert, of course. I will encourage them to relax and feel safe and get to know one another, tell their stories, and exchange telephone numbers.

I will drive to pick them up because they usually have no transportation unless someone offers it. I can do that. Maybe I can engage some of my age peers, women in their sixties and seventies, to help me. Or maybe they can host their own lunches. I envision doing it regularly, serving up social connection and a tenderly listening ear.

Launching the idea on Mother's Day weekend seems fitting, don't you think? It wouldn't have to be lunch—it could be an afternoon tea with home-made macaroons or angel cake and berries. Give those strawberries a dab of real whipped cream.

Recent research published in the British Medical Journal's publication *Heart* referenced twenty-three different studies done in Europe, Japan, Australia, and the United States. Researchers found that loneliness and social isolation have unanticipated and debilitating impacts on health and well-being, increasing the likelihood of heart disease and stroke by fifty percent. The studies looked at women (and men) who had limited social networks or supports, infrequent or poor quality social contact and feelings of isolation. The findings were so powerful that one headline refers to loneliness as "the new smoking."

I have written about this before. Sometimes certain newspaper columns I have written in the past generate broad-based feedback.

I hear things like, "I sent your last column to my sister in Alaska" or "That column of yours was a real call to action for me." But when I write about the health crisis presented by lonely and neglected elders, I cannot seem to create much of a buzz.

So I am trying a new approach. I will attempt to leverage any assuredly-existing Mother's Day sentiments. And I will do it now.

Let's start like this. We all had mothers. If yours is no longer with you, identify an elderly person who needs a ride, a few strawberries, or an invitation to get together for a friendly chat. It should not take you long—they are everywhere. So many aging women (and men) live alone, abandoned by distant relatives and forgotten by family who really never knew them in the first place.

If your mother is still with you, cherish her mightily, and if she is nearby, ask her to co-host a little luncheon get-together sometime in the next few weeks. Intermingle the generations. If she lives at a distance, when you call her today tell her about this idea. Thank you.

NOTES ON SOURCES

OLD LOVE

5   A 60-something author/activist: B. McDonald, *Making Sense of Women's Lives: An Introduction to Women's Studies* (Bowman and Littlefield, 2002)

5   I also thought about the poet: *M. Sarton, At Seventy: A Journal* (Open Road Media, 2014)

6   The presentation was titled: A. Nichols & S. Howard, "Gerontology Information and Training Needs of Cooperative Extension Professionals" (*Educational Gerontology* Vol 28. Issue 8, 2002)

7   What I want to explore: J. Sachs, *The Healing Power of Sex* (Prentice Hall, 1994)

7   There is research to show: D. Henes, *The Healing Power of Sex* (Huffington Post blog, February 13, 2013)

7   A Scottish study tried to figure it out: S.Brady "The Relative Benefits of Different Sexual Activity" (*Slate.com on-line post,* December 1, 2011)

11   It apparently changes as we age: O.Khazan, "The Dark Psychology of Being a Good Comedian" (*The Atlantic,* Feb 27, 2014)

13   I remember reading a book: M. Pipher, *Reviving Ophelia: Saving the Lives of Adolescent Girls* (Penguin Random House Audio, July 4, 2000)

14   I think the piece was titled something like: E. Bernstein, "Divorce's Guide to Marriage" (*Wall Street Journal,* July 24, 2012)

14   The importance of being more positive: T Orbuch, "The Early Years of Marriage Study" (University of Michigan EYM on-line newsletter, spring, 2009)

18   The rant starts out: M. Taraian, "Why the Festive Season Becomes Less Than Cheery" (*Odyssey on-line article,* Nov 21, 2017)

19   Nearly half of women over age: J. Beard et al. "Study: Older Women Living Longer but Gap between Rich and Poor Growing" (*World Health Organization on-line publication,* September 3, 2013)

23   The study was designed: S. Teshale & M.E. Lachman, "Managing Daily Happiness" (Brandeis University faculty publication, 2016)

FRIENDLIER AGING

29   When asked about the best terminology: J. Graham, "'Elderly' No More," (*New Old Age, New York Times on-line blog,* April 19, 2012)

32   A brief but rejuvenating aerobic work-out. M. Buchowski, "No Joke: Study Finds Laughter Burns Calories" (*Vanderbilt University Medical Center Weekly Newspaper*, June 10, 2005)

32   Go for more smiling behavior. J Rauch, "The Seven Types of Smiles and How People Perceive Them" (*Talkspace on-line blog*, October 12, 2015)

32   Apparently the psychologists: C. Kotchemidova, "To Smile or Not to Smile, The Evolution of Faces in Photos over 100 Years," (*University of California Berkeley publication*, December 1, 2005)

33   Experiment that used the recorded sounds of dogs laughing: S Coren, "Do Dogs Laugh?" (*Psychology Today on-line blog*, November 22, 2009)

35   I am uneasy about including them: K. McGlynn, "The 45 Funniest Autocorrect Fails of 2014" (*Huffington Post blog*, December 30, 2014)

42   But the real eye catcher was: P.R. Satran, "How Not to Act Old," (*Harper Collins*, 2009)

45   The comments from the sage: D. Hall, "The Poetry of Death" (*The New Yorker*, September 12, 2017)

44   Aging From a Peter Pan perspective: P. Turner, "Peter Pan, Alzheimer's Patient" (*The New Yorker*, December 24, 2012)

45   Well into old age himself: B.F. Skinner & M.E. Vaughn, "Enjoy Old Age: A Practical Guide," (*Amazon.com*, 1997)

46   Compliments are so important: G.Rubin, "The Power of Praise" (*Article in Good Housekeeping*, September 20, 2011)

46   In the words of the teacher-psychologist: H. Ginott, "Praise, Like Criticism Can Be Destructive," (*Facebook post*, November 19, 2015)

47   I just finished reading: J. Dideon, *The Year of Magical Thinking*, (Vintage International, 2007)

48   Keep functioning physically and psychologically: A. Sood et al, "SMART (Stress Management and Resiliency Training)," (*Mayo Clinic studies and publications*, 2017)

IDEAS THAT HEAL

52   The most referenced explanation: C. M. Aldwin & D.F.Gilmer, *Health, Illness and Optimal Aging*, (Sage Publications, 2004)

56   What they held in common: C. Kaiser, "'Broken Heart Syndrome Not Uncommon" (*Medpage Today*, July 19, 2011)

58   Research suggests: M.T. Brown & J.K. Bussell, "Medication Adherence: WHO Cares" (*Mayo Clinic Proceedings*, April. 2011)

60   You will assuredly follow their lead: B.J. Collingwood, "Researchers Tackle the Mystery of Yawning," (*Psych Central* blog, July 17, 2016)

60   There's a Theory: G.G. Gallup et al, "Yawning and Thermoregulation" (*Physiology and Behavior*, published on-line May 13, 2008)

61 Superstations about yawning abound: O. Walusinski et al, "Yawning: Comparative Study of Knowledge and Beliefs, Popular and Medical "(*Institute of Internal Medicine publication*, Madras Medical College, 2004)

62 Here's the bad news, really bad: J. A. Yanovski, "A Prospective Study of Holiday Weight Gain," (*NCBI-NIH Resources Public Access*, February 21, 2015)

62 There's an overwhelming association: J.A. Yanovski & N. Severing, *Living with Rheumatoid Arthritis*, (A Johns Hopkins Press Health Book, 2000)

64 Let me start at the beginning: N.M. Lambert "Expressing Gratitude to a Partner Leads to More Relationship Maintenance Behavior" (*PubMed*, February, 2011)

66 It was soundly ridiculed: R. Davis "The Man who Championed Handwashing and Briefly Saved Lives," (*Jefferson Public Radio Morning Edition*, January 12, 2015)

68 The source of these words: J.R.R. Tolkien, *The Hobbit*, (Houghton Mifflin Harcourt, 2012)

69 The original six-word story: C Constable, "Six Word Stories" (*Amazon Digital Services LLC*, 2012)

71 Did you sleep well last night: L. Epstein, "Twelve Simple Steps to Improve Your Sleep" (on-line article from the *Division of Sleep Medicine at Harvard Medical School*, December 18, 2007)

71 Here's my favorite approach: A. Pacivasek, "Study Uncovers Previously Unknown Molecular Bridge between Sleep and Memory" (*University of Maryland School of Medicine announcement*, September 28, 2017)

72 I may have a solution for you: M. Kondo, *The Life-Changing Magic of Tidying Up: The Japanese Art of Decluttering* (Ten Speed Press, 2014)

75 Sometimes we become totally smitten: D. Rotman, "Who Will Own the Robots" (*MIT Technology Review*, June 16, 2015)

AGING IN PLACE: GET READY

80 Such staying power we have: R. Adelson, *Staying Power: Age-Proof Your Home for Comfort, Safety and Style* (Sage Tree Publications, 2013)

82 They develop a fear of losing stability: Select authors, National Council on Aging, "Falls Free: Promoting a National Council on Aging Action Plan" (*NCOA publication*, 2005)

85 In a large sample of older adults: H. Chang, C. Lynm & R.M. Glass, "Falls and Older Adults" (*JAMA Network, JAMA Patient Page*, January 20, 2010)

86 Each hospitalized fall costs: "Important Facts about Falls" (*Centers for Disease Control (CDC) website*, February 10, 2017)

86 A fall expert: J. Schwartz & "Take Care" staff, "The Right Way to Fall: Preventing and Reducing Fall-Related Injuries" (*WRVO Public Media*, May 13, 2017)

89 Scholarly articles regularly report: R. Schwarzer & A. Luszczynska, "How to Overcome Health-Compromising Behaviors" (*Hogrefe and Hober Publishers*, 2008)

90   The beginning of an idea: S. Szanton, "Community Aging in Place—Advancing Better Living for Elders (CAPABLE)" (*Johns Hopkins University School Nursing on-line video,* 2015)

90   Here is another example: S.L. Szanton et al, "Medicaid Cost Savings of a Preventive Home Visit for Older Adults" (Journal of the American Geriatrics Society, Nov, 2017)

93   Healthy people are more productive: K. Lorig et al, *Living a Healthy Life with Chronic Conditions,* (Bull Publishing, 2018)

WHAT IF YOU DON'T REMEMBER WHAT YOU FORGOT?

100   Some degree of simple forgetting: Johns Hopkins University researchers and staff, "Guide to Memory Loss and Aging" (*Johns Hopkins Special Report/Health Alert,* 2009)

101   It caught my eye years ago: R. Sapolsky, "Depression in the U.S." (*Stanford University on-line video lecture,* November 10, 2009)

102   A very credible multi-year study: N.L van der Zwaluw et al, "Folate and Vitamin B12—Related Biomarkers in Relation to Brian Volumes" (*U.S. National Library of Medicine publication,* December 24, 2016)

102   A long-ago article: American Psychological Association (APA) staff writers, "Memory Changes in Older Adults" (*APA website,* June 11, 2006)

104   Here's an illustration: S. A. Cusack & W. Thompson, *Mental Fitness for Life: 7 Steps to Healthy Aging (Bull Publishing,* 2005)

105   Understanding what gives us the most trouble can be useful: V.O. Leirer et al., "Memory Skills Elders Want to Improve" (*Experimental Aging Research,* September 28, 2007)

106   Didn't I already know this: F.I. M. Craik, "Effects of Distraction and Memory on Cognition: A Commentary" (*Frontiers in Psychology,* July 29, 2014)

107   Address aging cognition in plain speak: K. J. Hsu, "Experimentally Induced Distraction Impacts Cognitive but Not Emotional Processes in Think-Aloud Cognitive Assessment" (*Frontiers in Psychology,* May 20, 2014)

108   Or even the roman room technique: A. Frakt, "An Ancient and Proven Way to Improve Memorization: Go Ahead and Try It" (*The Upshot,* New York Times, May 24, 2016)

110   Aging patients with chronic medical conditions: S.R. Brown, "The Why and How of High-Value Prescribing" (*American Family Physician,* February 15, 2016)

114   Think of your brain as plastic: B Strauch, "How to Train the Aging Brain" (*Education Life, New York Times,* December 29, 2009)

116   But wait: A.L. Murad, "15 Simple Diet Tweaks That Could Cut Your Alzheimer's Risk" (*Mayo Clinic on-line article,* August 17, 2017)

116   Research in the newsletter: Nutrition Action Newsletter staff, "Latest Expert Advice about Preventing Cognitive Decline and Dementia" (*Center for Science in the Public Interest,* July 6, 2017)

117   What a finding: J.A. Luchsinger, "Type 2 Diabetes, Related Conditions, in Relation and Dementia: An Opportunity for Prevention" (*Columbia University,* 2010)

ENGAGING SADNESS

120   Did you know: M. Trudeau "Human Connections Start with a Friendly Touch," (*NPR Morning Edition,* September 20, 2010)

120   Give it a try yourself: K. Menehan, "Tiffany Field on Massage Research" (*Massage Magazine,* January 2006)

122   I have lost myself: J. Gaugler et al, "2016 Alzheimer's Disease Facts and Figures" (*Published Report by the Alzheimer's Association,* 2016)

124   More likely to r-occur without treatment: "Depression Facts, Statistics and Figures" (*NIMH/ Healthline Newsletter,* January 28, 2015)

124   It is highly treatable: Mayo Clinic staff, "Depression" (*Mayo Clinic Patient Care and Health Information website,* February 3, 2018)

125   Depression is more subtle in the older adult: K. Duckworth,"Depression in the Older Adult" (*National Alliance on Mental Illness Fact Sheet,* October, 2009)

127   A well-written article: B. Briggs. "Get Off My Lawn! Why Some Older Men Get So Grouchy" (*Men's Health on NBC News,* December 28, 2012)

128   Your reaction when I'm done: Harvard Health Letter staff, "Insider Tips to Maximize Your Health Visit" (*Harvard Health Letter Publishing,* February, 2018)

130   Well-researched article: A. Walker et al. *Families in Later Life: Connections and Transitions* (Sage Publishing, 2001)

134   Is this the future of medical care: L. Zimmerman, "Hood: Trailblazer of the Genome Age" (*Amazon Digital LLC,* 2016)

136   A study done: L. Baker, "Pet-Owning Couples are Closer, Interact More than Pet-Less Couples" (*News Center, University of Buffalo,* March 12, 1998)

136   A study done: A.P. Shojai. "The Health Benefits of Pets" (*Huffington Post blog,* May 26, 2011)

138   Science may determine whether you're correct: B. Flamm, "The Columbia University 'Miracle' Study Flawed and Fraud" (*Skeptical Inquirer* September/October, 2004)

138   Prayer on behalf of cardiac patients: C Soares, "No Prayer Prescription" (*Scientific American,* June 19, 2006)

138   Replaced by systematic investigation: C. Andrade & R. Radhakrishan, "Prayer and Healing: A Medical and Scientific Perspective on Randomized, Controlled Trials" (*Indian Journal of Psychiatry,* October-December, 2009)

139   What's going on and why: M. Krucoff and Duke Today staff, "Prayer and Healing" (*Duke Today, Duke University on-line article,* November 30, 2001)

144 You probably know the reason: J. Hurley & B. Lieberman, "BIG: Movie Theaters Fill Bucket . . . and Bellies" (*Center for Science in the Public Interest,* December, 2009)

147 I stand in awe, completely: C. Seidenberg, "Spices and Their Health Benefits," (*Washington Post Wellness Section,* January 7, 2014)

148 That's what this message is all about: U. S. Food and Drug Administration staff, "Food Safety for Older Adults" (*FDA website,* November 8, 2017)

150 Celebration over: M. Guiliano, *The French Women Don't Get Fat: The Secret of Eating for Pleasure,* (Vintage, 2007)

152 Taste buds change as we age: M.Y. Park, "How Our Sense of Taste Changes as We Age" (*Bon Appetit Magazine,* May 14, 2014)

155 There's more: R. Fitzsimmons, "Oh, What Those Oats Can Do. Quaker Oats, the Food and Drug Administration and the Market Value of Scientific Evidence 1984-2010," (*Comprehensive Reviews in Food Science and Food Safety,* 2012)

157 A newspaper article titled: G. Taubes, "Is Sugar Toxic?" (*New York Times Magazine,* April 13, 2011)

157 The author takes a compelling look: G. Taubes, *Why We Get Fat and What to Do About It* (Anchor, 2011)

157 What you eat for lunch today: J. Calderone, "FDA Is Not So Sweet on Sugars" (*Consumer Reports,* June 1, 2016)

157 Some researchers believe sugar is poison: Y. Wei & M.J. Pagliassotti, "Hepatospecific Effects of Fructose on C-Jun NH2-Terminal Kinase: Implications for Hepatic Insulin Resistance" (*Pub Med,* November 28, 2004)

159 More impressive than almost any fruit I've encountered: "Mango Nutrition—Tropical Fruit for Lowering Blood Sugar and Boosting Brain Health" *Dr. Axe Food and Medicine website,* (July 20, 2015)

FAMILY FACTS AND FABLES

169 A regular feature titled: M. Atwood, "Margaret Atwood: By the Book," (*New York Times Book Review,* November 25, 2015)

169 In his book: W. Berger, *A More Beautiful Question: The Power of Inquiry to Spark Breakthrough Ideas* (Bloomsbury USA, 2016)

170 Vancouver Auditorium Education series, "Sea Otters: A Natural History," (*Live-streamed Resource Video Lecture,* October 16, 2014)

171 See the parallels here: R Davidson, "The Power of Holding Hands: A Study on Reducing Fear and Pain" (*Health and Well-Being Magazine,* September 5, 2010)

171 One that exudes warmth and caring: M. Hertenstein, "Power of Touch" (*NPR Morning Edition,* September 20, 2010)

176   An epidemiological study: J. Hammond & J. Brooks, "World Trade Center Attack: Helping the Helpers" (*U.S. National Library of Medicine, NIH,* November 6, 2001)

GIVING CARE

182   Open-mouthed while reading: H. Cisneros et al, *Independent for Life: Homes and Neighborhoods for an Aging America* (Texas University Press, 2012)

183   Aging experts tell us: N.R Nicholson Jr. "The Relationship between Injurious Falls, Fear of Falling, Social Isolation and Depression" (*University of Connecticut student theses,* June 2005)

183   Measurably healthier. J. Holt-Lunstad et al., "Social Relationships and Mortality Risk: A Meta-analytic Review" *(PLOS Medicine,* July 27, 2010)

184   Imagine this: K. Lorig et al., "Effect of a Self-Management Program on Persons with Chronic Disease" (*Effective Clinical Practice,* November/December 2001)

187   The site references: AARP Research Group, "The AARP Grandparenting Survey: The Sharing and Caring Between Mature Grandparents and their Grandchildren" (*AARP,* November 1999)

189   Other phrases that linger as well: S. de Toledo & D.E. Brown, *Grandparents as Parents: A Survival Guide for Raising a Second Family* (Guilford Press, 2013)

190   The somewhat less known author: L. Kessler, *Dancing with Rose or Finding Life in the Land of Alzheimer's: One Daughter's Hopeful Story* (Penguin Books, 2008)

192   As I recall it said something like: R.M. Leipzig, "The Patients Doctors Don't Know" (*New York Time Op Ed,* July 1, 2009)

193   I have found a few things that give me hope: R.M. Leipzig et al., "Consensus on AAMC Minimum Geriatric Competencies for Medical Students" (*Academic Medicine* July 1, 2009),

197   An on-line article: B. King, *The Laughing Cure: Emotional and Physical Healing—A Comedian Reveals Why Laughter Really is the Best Medicine* (Skyhorse Publishing, 2016)

197   Another on-line article: G. Barreca, "20 Rules That Everyone Can Live By" (*Psychology Today,* May 29, 2016)

198   Recent research published: N.K. Valtorta et al., "Loneliness and Isolation as Risk Factors for Coronary Artery Disease and Stroke: Systematic Review and Meta-analysis of Longitudinal Observational Studies" (*British Medical Journal,* HEART, April 18, 2016)

ABOUT THE AUTHOR

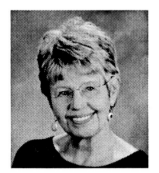 Sharon Johnson is an Oregon State University Associate Professor Emeritus. She has a Master's Degree in Rehabilitation and a Certificate in Gerontology from the University of Washington. She is a Certified Aging-in-Place Specialist (CAPS) through the National Association of Home Builders. In addition to her 12-year career at Oregon State University, Sharon served as the Deputy and Interim Director of the Seattle/King County Department of Public Health and was Washington State's Director of their Division of Mental Health.

Sharon lives with her husband, Howard, and their dog, "Lucille Ball," in the Rogue Valley of southern Oregon where she has written a well-received weekly Sunday column, *Healthy Aging* for over 15 years. After retirement, Sharon and Howard launched a non-profit organization and developed "Grandma's Porch," and a fall-risk assessment process that assists low-income elders in identifying in-home risks for fall and fracture and provides a talent pool of handymen (and women) to make needed home modifications (bathroom grab bars, shower benches, better lighting, secured scatter rugs) that keep elders safer at home. Grandma's Porch is funded by local foundations.

All proceeds from the purchase of *How Gray is My Valley* go to Grandma's Porch.